HUMAN
MULTIPLE REPRODUCTION

HUMAN
MULTIPLE REPRODUCTION

Ian MacGillivray
P. P. S. Nylander
Gerald Corney

with contributions by

Valerie Farr
E. B. Robson

1975

W. B. Saunders Company Ltd London · Philadelphia · Toronto

W. B. Saunders Company Ltd: 12 Dyott Street
London WC1A 1DB

West Washington Square
Philadelphia, Pa. 19105

833 Oxford Street
Toronto, Ontario M8Z 5T9

Library of Congress Cataloging in Publication Data
MacGillivray, Ian.
  Human multiple reproduction.

  1. Birth, Multiple. I Corney, G., joint
author. II. Nylander, Percy Palgrave Shaftesbury,
joint author. [DNLM: 1. Pregnancy, Multiple.
2. Twins. WQ235 M145h] III. Title.
RG696.M3   618.2'5   75—21750
ISBN 0-7216-5974-8

Printed by Billing & Sons Limited, Guildford and London

Print No: 9 8 7 6 5 4 3 2 1

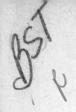

Contributors

G. CORNEY, MD, *Member of Scientific Staff, MRC Human Biochemical Genetics Unit, The Galton Laboratory, University College, London.*

V. FARR, MD, *Clinical Lecturer in Obstetrics and Gynaecology, University of Aberdeen; Medical Assistant (Ultrasonics and Perinatology), Aberdeen Maternity Hospital and Aberdeen Royal Infirmary, Aberdeen.*

I. MACGILLIVRAY, MD, FRCP, FRCOG, *Regius Professor of Obstetrics and Gynaecology, University of Aberdeen; Consultant Obstetrician/Gynaecologist, Aberdeen Maternity Hospital and Aberdeen Royal Infirmary, Aberdeen.*

P. P. S. NYLANDER, MB, ChB, MRCP(Ed.), FRCOG, *Professor and Head, Department of Obstetrics and Gynaecology, University College Hospital, Ibadan, Nigeria; Consultant Obstetrician and Gynaecologist, University College Hospital, Ibadan, Nigeria.*

E. B. ROBSON, PhD, *Assistant Director, MRC Human Biochemical Genetics Unit, University College, London.*

Contents

Preface

Many books have been published on multiple births in humans. They deal with different individual aspects; for example, Scheinfeld (1973) and Mittler (1971) on the behavioural aspects, Strong and Corney (1967) on placentation, Gedda (1961) on the history of twinning and Bulmer (1970) on zygosity, genetics and incidence. There is a need, however, for a comprehensive book dealing with most of these aspects which would be of interest to the obstetrician, paediatrician, physiologist, geneticist, human reproductive biologist or the interested midwife or medical student. This book does not attempt to cover all the aspects in detail, but ample references have been given for more extensive reading.

The authors have collaborated in writing this book because of their interest in different aspects of twinning, as will be apparent from their contributions. The main original work quoted by the authors was done in Nigeria, Aberdeen and Oxford. It is somewhat prophetic that it was a hundred years ago that a connection between Aberdeen and twinning in Nigeria took place in another way. It was in May 1875 that Mary Slessor, who was born in Aberdeen, went to Calabar, Nigeria, to the mission field and was responsible for saving many of the twins either rejected or in danger of being killed because of taboos (Christian and Plummer, 1970). The high incidence of twinning in Nigeria was probably not only responsible for those taboos, but also for stimulating the interest in the causation of twins, and indeed, for the production of this book.

We wish to thank our publishers for their understanding and help, Mr E. Smith, Medical Illustration Department, Medical School, University of Aberdeen, for his excellent illustrations, and also Mr A. J. Lee, University College, London, for Figures 3.10 and 3.11. Special acknowledgement is given to Mrs D. Seedburgh, University College, London, for researching much of the detail in Chapter 1, and to all those who have helped either in the original work contained in this book or in the preparation of this manuscript.

I. MACGILLIVRAY
P. P. S. NYLANDER
G. CORNEY

1975

CHAPTER 1

Mythology and Customs Associated with Twins

G. CORNEY

In the closing decades of the twentieth century, the simultaneous birth of two or more infants gives rise to little, or at most transitory excitement or wonder in most communities and such multiple births have increasingly become accepted as a normal variation in the outcome of conception and subsequent pregnancy. This has not always been the case however and most, if not all societies at some stage in their evolution have probably regarded such births with a mixture of awe and fear. As a consequence elaborate legends, cults and ceremonies associated with twins are commonly found in the histories of many societies, though these beliefs and customs must have arisen in the absence of any knowledge of the biological aspects of the situation, as detailed scientific information on monozygotic and dizygotic twinning has only been available during the last hundred years. The immense number of myths and customs which can be found in association with the delivery of twins probably arose simply because, inexplicably, two babies arrived when one was expected. Though this situation was accepted as normal for animals, it must have seemed extremely abnormal for human beings and therefore the community had to devise ways to help everyone adjust to this threatening event.

This phenomenon of ritual and taboos associated with twin births seems to have been worldwide and presumably has considerable social anthropological significance. Reference to the matter is quite common, but this is often to be found, as might be expected, scattered throughout books on particular ethnic groups or geographical areas. However, there are two monographs on the topic, namely those of Harris (1913) and of Lagercrantz (1941). The former deals with the whole subject, the latter being mainly confined to customs in Africa. Other useful sources are the various encyclopaedias of folklore and customs; one of these contains the very comprehensive review of Hartland (1921). The question is also discussed by Gedda (1961) and Scheinfeld (1973).

In this chapter a brief general survey of mythology and rituals associated with twinning throughout the world will be given but particular emphasis will be placed on the African continent as customs there seem to be particularly well documented. Many of the customs are similar in different societies but a few will be discussed in detail to illustrate the various social attitudes and methods of expressing them.

MYTHOLOGY

Twins figure quite prominently in the mythology of the ancient cultures of Rome and Greece. Romulus and Remus were the sons of Mars, their mother being Sylvia, a Vestal Virgin who was condemned to be drowned in the Tiber with her twin children. As is well known, this evil plan had an unexpected outcome as the cradle containing the twins became stranded, the twins were cared for and suckled by a she-wolf and subsequently found by a shepherd. In later life they decided to found a city on the banks of the Tiber, but strife arose over the choice of a site and Remus was killed by his brother after a quarrel. He therefore never saw the city of Rome over which Romulus ruled for many years.

Amongst the most famous, however, were Castor and Pollux. They were worshipped in Greece, Sicily and Italy, especially as guardians of seafarers, Poseidon (Neptune) having rewarded their brotherly love by giving them power over the wind and the waves. Their safe guidance in rough storms was sometimes associated with a strange light often known as *St. Elmo's fire*. Castor was killed in a battle but Pollux survived. Solitary existence on earth was not an attractive proposition for Pollux, who pleaded with Zeus for permission to join his brother in the heavens. The solution to this dilemma is variously reported, but some say that the brothers were allowed days alternately on Earth and with the gods on Mount Olympus: other versions give them eternal peace as stars (*Gemini*) in the heavenly constellation (Smith, 1853; Harris, 1913, 1928; Gedda, 1961; Allegro, 1970).

The Dioscuri (referred to as *Castores* by the Romans) played a significant role in both Greek and Roman mythology, but a wider influence known as *Dioscurism* has been suggested. The significance of this in Indo-European mythology and its implications for other civilisations have been studied extensively by Harris (1913) and others (Leach, 1949). Comparisons have been made between the two Açvins or Celestial Horsemen in the *Rig-Veda* from India, twins in European mythologies and customs in many other parts of the world, especially Africa.

There is now often very little overt trace of these original beliefs in the social life of the various communities, but evidence of them can usually be found in the appropriate literature, paintings or statuary. As an illustration it is useful to review customs in different countries, particularly in Africa where attitudes showed great variation (Hartland, 1921) even within a relatively small geographical area.

ATTITUDES TOWARDS TWINS IN VARIOUS COUNTRIES

EUROPE

Records of customs in Western Europe (Harris, 1913; Hartland, 1921) deal largely with folklore attached to twins without giving any clue as to the real attitude of society towards them. At the present time, apart from mild curiosity, this might be said to be neutral. But evidently this was not always the case, as in mediaeval Europe the mother was thought to have been unfaithful to her husband because twins implied two fathers (Giles, 1908). Water from the well of St. Mungo in Scotland, if taken by the tumblerful, was said to ensure a subsequent twin birth but the ever-cautious Scotswomen dealt with this myth by taking only half a glass of water from the well! In both Scotland and England it was believed that infertility would follow a twin-birth and also that the twins themselves might be childless. It was also considered that twins would die within short periods of each other; however, if one did survive longer, then the 'left twin' was (in Sussex) credited with healing powers, particularly for thrush in the mouth (Rorie, 1914; Radford and Radford, 1961). As recently as the early part of this century twins were associated with good luck and fertile influences in Wales and were apparently in demand to attend marriages there, thus ensuring luck to the wedded pair. At weddings in Bulgaria the mothers of bride and groom simultaneously drank brandy as this alcoholic union of mothers-in-law was thought to prevent twin grandchildren.

In Brittany two apples preserved in a hollow oak and representing the children of thunder were thought to be able to quell a storm and, also in France, women who ate double nuts or fruit would, it was felt, subsequently have twins. In mediaeval France, twins could evidently be associated with curses and banishment. An altar found in Notre Dame contained a dedication to Celtic Deities including Heavenly Twins. Excavations in Belgium have revealed pairs of small funeral urns within a larger one thought to date back to the Iron Age and it has been suggested that the custom of twin-murder might have prevailed in Belgium in prehistoric times. In Eastern Europe in the region of the Carpathian Mountains the Huzuls believed that the birth of twins implied early death of the parents, a belief similar to that expressed in territories as far apart as South Africa and Indonesia.

ASIA AND THE FAR EAST

Information is much more scanty with regard to attitudes to twins in these areas, in some parts of which twin birth rates happen to be very low, due to the small numbers of dizygotic twins (Bulmer, 1970). In Japan, though little information is available and reports are inconsistent, it would seem that twin births were at one time viewed with distaste, certainly in some areas. This would seem anomalous to those who hold the view that aversion to multiple births was found only in more primitive civilisations. Information about a twin birth was often suppressed there and amongst the nobility one of the twins was given away to a courtier. The fact that the baby had been a twin was however recorded as, should the other twin die, he could then be returned to court (Veith, 1960). It would not therefore seem that the low rate of twinning in these parts necessarily meant that twins were any more favourably regarded. In Northern Japan, the Giljakē and Ainu people looked upon twin births with some awe and fear because it was believed that a spirit was the father of one of them, but which member of the pair had spiritual paternity was uncertain. Whether twins were killed or not in these areas is in dispute, but certainly attempts were made to conceal such a birth because of the subsequent disrepute which would fall upon the family. However, the family would present offerings to the twins, build little huts for them and also make images. If one twin did die, the Saghalien Ainu then identified him as the one with the spirit-father (Harris, 1913). The Tungus of Manchuria detested twins and would not allow anything to be borrowed or bought from their mother lest the calamity should then fall upon others (Webster, 1942).

Pacific islands

The Bontoc Igorot and Ifugoas of Luzon in the Philippines allowed only one twin to live (Webster, 1942; Barton, 1946) as did the Kayans in Borneo. The motive amongst the latter was that the death of one would preserve the life of the other, as he or she would not then have to share the milk and would also be less liable to sickness because, in view of a sympathetic bond between twins, each was thought to be susceptible to the illnesses of the other (Hose and McDougall, 1912). In the Solomon Islands one twin was usually killed and in Melanesia it was the custom to kill either one or both, the decision resting with the mother (Pitt-Rivers, 1914; Webster, 1942). The sex of the twins determined their fate in New Britain; both were allowed to live if they were of the same sex, but if not, then the girl was killed. Twins were accepted in Samoa, however, though triplets were disliked (Brown, 1910). It was believed by the Mundugumor in New Guinea that twins might result if the husband had intercourse with his wife after she was known to be pregnant. Both were allowed to live if they were female, but if twins were of different sex, the boy might not be kept. However, one member of the pair was always adopted as the women would not undertake to suckle two children (Mead, 1939).

AUSTRALIA

Amongst the Australian Aboriginals one twin was said to be the result of witchcraft from evil spirits and might therefore contaminate others and possibly betray tribal secrets when he grew up. The suspect one was therefore destroyed, usually by one of the old women in attendance (Spencer and Gillen, 1899; Basedow, 1925). This abhorrence of twins (sanctions apparently were not expressed against the mother) was prevalent in Northern, Central and South-Eastern Australia. The explanation that twins were hard to rear because there was not enough food for both does not seem adequate as the same customs were found when food was plentiful. It would seem more likely that the attitude was again an expression of the dread of the abnormal, in this case taking the form of anger that the spirits had given the mother something so strange to rear (Harris, 1913).

ESKIMOS

When twins are born, the Eskimos formerly killed at least one. Alternatively the infant might be adopted by another family as it was not thought possible for a mother to care for both in conditions of such hardship (Weyer, 1932).

AFRICA

Though customs were associated with twinning all over the world, they were particularly common and extremely varied in type in Africa (Hartland, 1921; Loeb, 1958; Jeffreys, 1963). Harris (1913) in his monograph 'Boanerges' (*Sons of Thunder*) deals with many aspects of the twin cult and records that taboos with regard to twins were reported from Nigeria as early as the mid-seventeenth century, though there was considerable dispute as to some of the sources of information. There were however numerous reports during the next two hundred years from travellers to West Africa in particular. The general theme was that twins and their mothers were regarded as hardly human, possibly by comparison with multiple-bearing lower animals. Both mother and children were therefore often destroyed and the abhorrence was such that even the area surrounding the birth (or burial) place of the twins was looked upon as desecrated ground. These early reports were naturally somewhat limited in geographical terms, but there was evidence, amply confirmed in more recent times, that the reaction to a double birth was by no means always the same in one area or within the same tribe. One might therefore have a mother and her twins killed or greatly revered in communities which were only separated by a relatively short distance. The reason for this is still not completely understood. The modes of expressing sanctions were however very diverse and it would therefore be worth reviewing both the more general aspects of the twin-reaction and in addition some individual customs, such as the cult of twin images, in particular the Ibeji statues in Nigeria, the use of *fixed names* and also the influence that twins were thought to have on the weather.

One can record the areas in which twins were *welcome* and *unwelcome* and this particular aspect amongst various tribes on the African continent is dealt with by Lagercrantz (1941) who illustrates his monograph with diagrams indicating the distribution of various customs. As has already been mentioned, the situation is very confusing to assess, even in a relatively small part of such a large and culturally diverse continent. The situation in Nigeria, as shown diagrammatically in Figure 1.1, serves to illustrate the diversity of the reaction, an example being the small area west of Lagos in which the Egun (or

Popo) peoples welcomed twins (Chappel, 1974) in contrast to the major part of Yorubaland.

Violent aversion to twins seems to have been due to one or other, or possibly a combination of, two main beliefs:

1. that as multiple births occur in lower animals, by analogy, human twins and their mother (and possibly, though much less commonly voiced, their father) should be regarded as such and were therefore unfit to exist;

2. that there was a problem of paternity as two infants must mean that there had been two fathers. Thus the mother must have been unfaithful and had intercourse either with a man other than her husband, or with an evil spirit. In either circumstance it would mean that she had been defiled and such

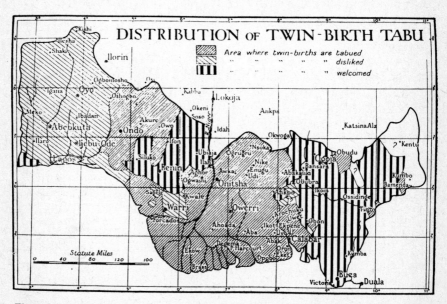

Figure 1.1. The distribution of twin-birth tabu in Southern Nigeria. From Talbot, P. A. *The Peoples of Southern Nigeria*, Vol. 3, published by Oxford University Press, London (1926), with permission.

paternity disputes provided grounds for the disturbance of peace and stability of the whole society.

Whatever the correct explanation in a particular community, the inescapable conclusion was that the land, the community and the mother must be purified and elaborate rituals were devised for this purpose. In terms of the general community or the land, the sanction in its most severe form was for the twins and the mother to be killed. In less stringent form the mother was banished from the community to the bush, or *twin-towns* (Leonard, 1906; Harris, 1913) might be created for such mothers and they would only be allowed back after a specified period. In general the father was free from guilt, possibly because of confusion over the dual paternity theory. The degree of revulsion with which twin births were regarded can be assessed from the terrible curses which could be delivered in the context of twins; these might be verbal, thus the curse *nam-a-shoobra*, meaning 'one of twins' or 'half a man' was regarded as a terrible curse when delivered by a chief, but words were not always necessary to convey malice. The same effect could be achieved in silence if the right arm with two fingers outstretched was raised in the direction of a woman, it conveyed the terrifying message 'may you become the mother of twins' (deCardi, 1899; Lagercrantz, 1941).

Contact with other people, as with the arrival of missionaries such as Mary Slessor in Calabar, Nigeria (Christian and Plummer, 1970), led to greater social and scientific understanding with subsequent modification of sanctions of this type. That this process was far from simple is however demonstrated by two reports of legal trials with regard to ritual twin murders in South Africa. The first (Harris, 1913) happened in 1910 amongst the Matabele, the parents being subsequently brought to trial at the Circuit Court in Bulawayo. The death sentence was pronounced, but later reduced to penal servitude. The second, over ten years later, concerned Basuto (or Makalala) parents in Bechuanaland. In the latter case the death penalty was also imposed by the court, but later commuted by the High Commissioner to imprisonment with hard labour for five years. In both these cases, however, one had an anomalous situation in which the complex legal system of one society was passing judgement on the long-standing tribal customs of another. The court would not accept their plea that if the white men would guarantee no harm would follow, such traditional customs would be abandoned. It would have been difficult for a colonial judge to estimate the intensity of primal fear which might have led to such a twin-murder, despite the fact that the ancestors of his own society almost certainly exhibited similar taboos (Harris, 1922). Confusion might also arise within a tribe as amongst the Samburu in Kenya (Spencer, 1965) if one member disregards the taboo and, contrary to predictions, continues to prosper.

Modifications of such sanctions might well begin with those towards the mother (Harris, 1913). Evidence of changing attitudes to ritual ceremonies surrounding a twin birth might also be found in the lack of enthusiasm amongst younger members of a society for the traditional customs of their elders (Wagner, 1936). Gradually, therefore, taboos would become less pronounced and subsequently disappear through the generations. Complete reversal of earlier practices might also occur as in the case of the Yoruba in West Africa who now welcome twins but, according to many authorities, practised sanctions against them in earlier times (Chappel, 1974).

PARTICULAR CUSTOMS ASSOCIATED WITH TWINS

TWIN IMAGES

The use of images in association with twins, most frequently as a substitute for one who had died, is common in Africa, particularly tropical Africa (Lagercrantz, 1941). Such statues were reported by early explorers to the continent and in 1862, Speke, on his return journey through Uganda after discovering the source of the Nile, was told of a Myoro woman who kept two pots in her house as effigies of her dead twins. It was the custom for the mother to put her milk into these for five months, as that was thought to be the natural period for suckling children. In another province he heard that the mother of a dead twin would tie a small gourd round her neck into which she placed a trifle of everything given to the living child, lest she should be tormented by the dead spirit (Speke, 1863). The most extensive use of effigies seems, however, to be found in the Ibeji cult amongst the Yorubas of South-Western Nigeria. The word *ibeji* (to beget two) is used in Yoruba either as a general name for twins or for the deity (*Orisha*) of twins (Abraham, 1958). A temple dedicated to this god was situated between Lagos and Badagry and it was customary for twins and their parents to make a pilgrimage there. The same word is also used for the wooden image customarily carved after the death of one twin, the intention being either to provide company for the survivor or to give the spirit of the deceased a refuge (Ellis, 1894). The use of the Ibeji statues and the Ibeji cult is discussed in a comprehensive review by Segy (1970). Although the use of carved wooden images of this type is widespread amongst the Yorubas of South-Western Nigeria, the custom is not universal in Africa as it has been estimated that amongst 200 tribes who welcome twins there, only about thirty make such effigies.

One reason for the prevalence of this type of statuary and associated customs amongst the Yorubas may well be attributable to their extremely high rate of twinning (Nylander, 1971b). This is probably the highest in the world and would, particularly in earlier times, certainly have been associated with a very high infant mortality. It has been suggested that this combination of a high rate of twin birth and death required a particular set of religio-social regulations and that this took the form of the Ibeji cult. Confirmation of this is found in the similar pattern of behaviour amongst the Yorubas to other anomalies such as albinos and dwarfs. Such mysterious and frightening aberrations from normal birth would, in the absence of scientific information, be inexplicable and responsibility was therefore placed on the *Orisha Ibeji*. Maintenance of a statue meant that the '*one-soul*' concept of the twins could be preserved and thus fear was in effect transformed into joy. The *babalawo* (priest) would prescribe an effigy to be carved from wood in the same sex as the deceased. Such images were usually carved after death, but this was not an invariable rule as a pair might be made soon after birth, though this was uncommon, as was the making of a pair after the death of both. If they were carved during life, then they bore the facial markings of the family (*abaja*) and were clothed similarly to the twins, being offered the same food. They might also be adorned with silver and jewellery (Figure 1.2). Segy (1970) discusses in considerable detail with many illustrations the various types of Ibeji statues with an analysis of particular features, including the elaborate hair-styles, which almost represent the signature of the carver. The average height is about ten inches. After the death of one twin, the statue would be carried by the mother as if it were a child, until such time as the surviving twin could take over this duty. He would then maintain this for the whole of his life. Much feasting would accompany these ceremonies, the mother always being greeted warmly as it was considered lucky to meet her. The statues were carefully cleaned, rubbed with oil (Sealey, 1973), clothed and given offerings such as kola nuts. They were given a special position in the family hut, and should a statue be sold, it was required that a new one should be made for the spirit of the deceased twin; the old figure then became 'soulless'.

Yoruba peoples living in Northern Nigeria also maintained the tradition of the doll-image which was there called *Asshe;* the mother believed that she would never give birth to another child if she did not have such an image. The twin gods (*Orisha Ibeji*) in Yoruba culture have been compared to the twin gods *Osiris* and *Ra* in ancient Egypt and this has been used as supporting evidence for the influence of Egyptian culture on that of other African peoples, though there is dispute about this (Loeb, 1958; Jeffreys, 1963).

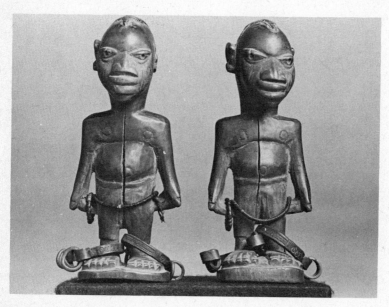

Figure 1.2. Nigerian wooden male figures carved in memory of twins. Courtesy of *The Illustrated London News*.

Evidence of the Ibeji cult can be found, however, in the Caribbean and in South America, where, as in Africa, there is a strong belief in the mystic significance of twins (Landes, 1940). In Cuba they are worshipped alongside the Catholic saints, St. Comas and St. Damien (Bascom, 1951). The culture is also found in Brazil (Verger, 1960) representing the transfer of culture by the Yoruba people imported as slaves. Bahia was the main port of entry of Negro slaves into Brazil, and as sugar cane became cultivated on a large scale huge numbers of slaves, as many as 100 000, arrived during the last twenty years of the eighteenth century (Frazier, 1942; Verger, 1968). Much of their culture, of which the *Ibeji* tradition is an example, still survives. This Yoruba ancestry also probably accounts for the relatively high dizygotic twinning rate found in Salvador, Brazil (Morton, 1970).

In Dahomey, the deity of twins is *Hoho* and a similar name (hohovi) is

given to twins. As in Nigeria, effigies are made (Figure 1.3) and it was customary for the carved image of a dead twin to be carried by the surviving one
(Ellis, 1894; Herskovits, 1938). There is evidence of similar statues being used
elsewhere in Africa, but the customs were not always consistent, for example
in Mali different names were used for male and female carvings and if the
surviving twin died, the original carving was thrown away (Segy, 1970).
Similar images or dolls have been reported from Togo and Angola (Stevenson, 1941a). In the Congo when a twin child died, a piece of wood was carved
into an image of the child and given to the survivor so that he would not be
lonely. Should he in turn die, then the effigy was buried with him (Hartland,
1921). In South-Eastern Africa the Ovimbundu make a figurine if one twin

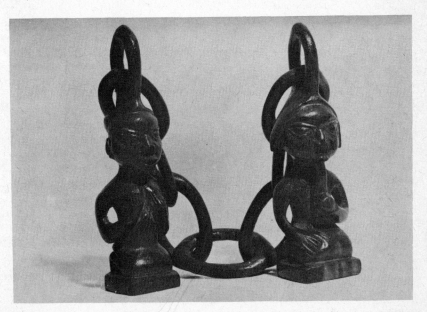

Figure 1.3. Wooden twin images from Dahomey, joined by seven links, all from one
piece of wood without joints. The male twin smokes a pipe. Courtesy of Professor E.G.
Parrinder.

dies, which is to prevent the other twin dying from loneliness; should the
survivor also die the effigy is buried with him (Hambly, 1937).

On the island of Nias (West of Sumatra), the father would ask the priest
to make a magical image, roughly human in shape, as an amulet against a
further twin birth (Hartland, 1921). Images of birds, fish and animals were
sometimes associated with twin births as, for example, amongst the Nutka
(or Nootka) of Vancouver Island who exhibited wooden images of birds and
fish around the hut in which twins had been born, thus extending an invitation
to birds and fish to visit them. The birth of twins was said to be an omen for a
good salmon year. There was a complex symbolism associating birds and
twins amongst the Nuer in the Sudan. These people had many beliefs relating
to twins, in particular that they had a single soul. In Asia the Kamchatkan

tribes set up a figure of a wolf made of grass (which was renewed yearly) after a twin birth in order to prevent a recurrence of such a strange event. The Giljakē, on the island of Saghalien in Northern Japan, feared the return of a dead twin and to counteract this, made a small hut containing an image to which food was taken each day (Harris, 1913; Hartland, 1921; Evans-Pritchard, 1936).

FIXED NAMES

Amongst a survey of African tribes (Segy, 1970), it has been found that at least 75 of them give *fixed names* to twins and some idea of the general distribution of this custom can be obtained from Figure 1.4. The practice is particularly prominent in Yoruba culture in Nigeria where the general name for twins, as has been described, is *Ibeji* ('to beget two'). However, amongst the several names traditionally given to a Yoruba child, those born in particular circumstances have a special (*amutọrunwa*) name and all other children born in similar circumstances are given the same name (Talbot, 1926a). In the case of twins, the first-born is called *Taiwo* (meaning 'he who has first taste of the world') an alternative being Ebo and the second is called *Kainde* or *Kehinde* ('he who lags behind') (Abraham, 1958; Segy, 1970). The first-born is considered to be the younger as he is sent in advance by the elder (and stronger) twin to announce his forthcoming birth and also to see if the world is a fit place for him (the elder brother) to enter. It is believed that if the first twin does not cry it will be difficult for the second to follow (Idowu, 1962). Another name which might be given to one of twin children is *Edon* or *Edun* after a small black monkey called *Edon dudu* or *Edun oriokum*, generally found amongst mangrove trees and said to be sacred to *Ibeji*, the deity of twins (Ellis, 1894). The child born subsequent to twins is called *Idowu* and is usually considered to be stubborn; however, any sacrifice offered for the twins must first be offered for the *Idowu*. Formerly, if these ceremonies were not carried out, it was considered that the twins might die (Abraham, 1958). In the case of triplets the third one is called *Idowu* (the servant of twins). The next child is *Alaba* (the servant of *Idowu*), the next again being *Idogbe* who watches the house whilst the others come, and is thought to be very precious. Other names indicative of seniority are given in Southern Nigeria, the elder twin being called *Odion* and the younger *Omo* (Thomas, 1919, 1921).

In Northern Nigeria, the Yergum give twin boys the names *Tali* and *Bali*. Amongst some tribes in the North, the ceremony for naming twins might be delayed, for example, the Kagoma custom is for a (single) child to be named by the eldest male member of the family within a day or two of birth, but in the case of twins this is not carried out until two months after the birth, when the ceremony is performed by the oldest man in the village. The Kaje and Jaba both delay the ceremony for twins until the seventh day when the child is named by the elders of the village instead of the parents as is customary (Temple, 1922; Meek, 1925).

In Dahomey, where twins (*hohovi*) are revered, there are special names for those children who follow the birth of the twins; the next child, if male, is called *Dósu*, if female, *Dosî*. The second after twins would be *Dósa* (male) or *Dóhwê* (female), and the third *Dónyŏ* (male) and *Dohwevî* (female). Not all these named groups are equally favoured though, as the *dósu* (child after twins) is to some extent disliked, being said to be avaricious, possessive and unreliable. Some other groups of favoured births, notably children born with the umbilical cord round the neck, feet foremost or in a caul, are regarded as twins from the point of view of appropriate ceremonies and are worshipped according to the rites of the twin cult known as *xoxo* (Herskovits, 1938; Mercier, 1954). In the Sudan the Nuer name the first child *Buth* (the one who precedes) and the second *Duoth* (the one who follows). Other names might be associated with seniority in the family or with birds (Evans-Pritchard, 1936).

WEATHER

In Egypt the twin gods *Shu* and *Tefnut* were regarded as twins shining as stars in the constellation of the heavens, Shu being the wind-god and Tefnut the sender of rain (Jeffreys, 1963). Similar attributions to the Heavenly Twins in Greek and Roman mythology (Frazer, 1905; Stevenson, 1941b) have been discussed previously. Power over the elements has also been bestowed on twins or circumstances surrounding their birth or death in countries as far apart as tropical Africa, North America and India (Hartland, 1921).

In the African continent such beliefs seem to be common in the East and South-East (Figure 1.4) but not apparently in West Africa (Harris, 1913). A creation myth amongst the Fon of Dahomey relates that there were primeval twins, *Mawu* (female) representing the Moon and living in the West, and *Lisa* (male), the Sun, living in the East. They are said to have come together at the time of an eclipse and were the parents of all other gods. These included the twin-gods of Storm who lived in the sky and had powers over thunder and lightning; further deities ruled the land, sea and the space between the earth and the sky (Mercier, 1954; Parrinder, 1967). Elsewhere in West Africa information is scanty; there is considerable general folklore in connection with thunder, lightning and rain in Southern Nigeria, which includes sky-deities (Talbot, 1926b), but there do not seem to be any legends or tribal customs associating twins and the weather in contrast to territories North and South of the Zambesi. Throughout Eastern and Southern Africa it was thought that the birth of twins did affect the climate and explorers such as Speke heard stories that twins were killed and thrown into water immediately after birth lest drought, famine or floods should oppress the land. Subsequently more details emerged indicating that such customs were widespread in the area (Speke, 1863; Hartland, 1921). There seemed to be a general feeling that after the birth of twins a period of mourning for the land was required with subsequent purification ceremonies before rain would fall again.

The Baronga in Mozambique gave the name of *Tilo* (the sky) to a woman who had given birth to twins, the infants being called 'the children of the sky'. In September and October, if the rains did not come, the women performed elaborate ceremonies such as cleansing all the local wells and subsequently pouring water over a mother of twins. The graves of twins might be given a similar drenching and if these graves were situated in a very dry area, they might be moved to the vicinity of a lake. The explanation is thought to be that by drenching the mother (who represented the sky) with water, the sky

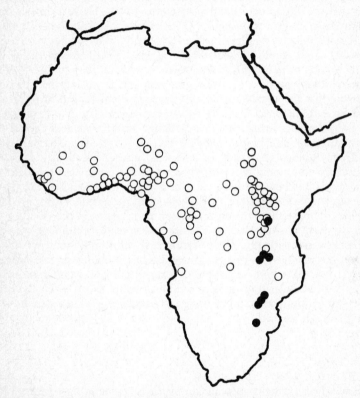

Figure 1.4. Map of Africa illustrating the distribution of *fixed names* for twins (open circles) and also customs associating twins and the weather (closed circles). Adapted from Lagercrantz (1941).

being saturated would then overflow and produce rain. Such ceremonies illustrate the former belief that anomalies of pregnancy, such as miscarriages or twin births, presaged disaster for the whole land if some form of purification ritual was not carried out. The Maluleke clan from an adjacent area of South-Eastern Africa believed that twins and other abnormal births should be cremated with an appropriate ceremony, the smoke from the funeral pyre constituting a religious offering. The country was then purified and rain would be expected to fall (Frazer, 1900; Junod, 1927; Dornan, 1932). Amongst the

Ama Xosa, twins were said to be able to divert a hailstorm by throwing a stone towards the storm, simultaneously shouting the direction to which the storm should go. A twin might be consulted by local people as his own state of health was thought to predict the weather, for example, if he was well it would not rain (Schapera, 1927).

Amongst North American Indians, the Mohave believed that twins came from the sky using lightning, thunder and rain as a means of descent. They were clad in wind, clouds and rain and could create thunder by rolling rocks about. Should lightning strike near to the house of a pregnant woman it was thought that she would bear twins (Devereux, 1941). There were a number of such myths amongst the Indians of British Columbia: the Skgomic thought twins had supernormal powers over the winds and if their bodies were rubbed with grease, winds would immediately arise; the Tsimshian prayed for wind and rain to abate by saying 'calm down breath of twins'; the Shuswap attributed to twins particular powers over rain and snow and the Thompson Indians held that the grizzly bear gave twins special powers including creation of good or bad weather. The Nootkas had a ceremony of darkening and washing the face to bring rain, the analogy being that rain would then drip from dark clouds (Frazer, 1900; Harris, 1913; Hartland, 1921). In South American mythology, brothers, often twins, appear frequently as culture heroes and are commonly represented as being diverse in strength, character and achievement. They are often identified with the Sun and the Moon and are given names which, in the various dialects, mean either Moon or Sun. Storms are attributable to quarrels between them and rain the result of beer spilt during their brawls! Such myths are widespread throughout the whole South American continent, some particularly intriguing such as the one regarding the twin heroes Amalivaca and Vochi who, after arranging for the surface of the earth to take on its present form, attempted to make the Orinoco flow simultaneously in both directions. This ingenious plan was devised to facilitate travel and the younger brother was blamed for the failure of the project (Métraux, 1946).

THE PLACENTA

In parts of Africa, some groups, including the Baganda in East Africa, looked upon a singleton placenta as the twin or double of the child (Hartland, 1921). The afterbirth was buried at the root of a plantain tree with some variation in ritual according to the sex of the child. Elaborate ceremonies were accorded to the afterbirth of a king. This was preserved in a special temple during his lifetime and a guardian was appointed who was given very high rank in the royal household. After the death of the monarch, his afterbirth remained in the charge of the newly appointed guardian in the court of his successor. Further south in Kiziba the afterbirth was considered as a human being and twins were therefore regarded as four children.

The Wanyoro kept the placenta in an earthen pot for which they built a special hut. After the death of the twins and a long period of mourning, the placentae and the twins were given a miniature hut. The Babangi placed the placentae on either side of a road or at crossroads, with a forked stick to mark the spot. This was decorated with coloured pots. Associations between the soul of a person and his afterbirth are also to be found amongst the Hausa in Northern Nigeria (Meek, 1937).

Similar beliefs were held in many of the islands in the Pacific and South China Seas and in addition the umbilical cord was occasionally, in Celebes, for example, treated as a further sibling (Long, 1963). Throughout Indonesia (Harris, 1913) special measures were often taken to guard the placenta during a person's lifetime. These were however withdrawn on his death when the soul of the placenta was united with that of the dead man and they were thus able to travel together to the realms of the dead.

CONCLUSION

Thus whilst the nature of customs associated with the birth of twins varied a great deal, the event seems universally to have represented a threat to the whole community. This was apparently a qualitative rather than a quantitative effect, as rituals were equally to be found in areas such as South-Western Nigeria where the twinning rate is very high and in the Far East where it is very low. These taboos probably derived from the reactions of people who were understandably frightened by this uncanny happening. The revulsion may have been due to a combination of emotions. A plural birth was thought to be (by comparison with animals) a degrading event for the mother, her family and the whole group. There was also the suspicion that the mother had been unfaithful either with another man or with an evil spirit. Economy of food supplies as a reason for adoption or slaughter of one of the twins probably constituted only a convenient explanation which masked these more primitive beliefs (Devereux, 1960). A further problem was the difficulty of accepting two people of the same age into a society in which seniority was of great importance in the social structure. A solution was the destruction of one or both twins or, as with the Nuer in the Sudan, giving them a single personality (Schapera, 1927; Evans-Pritchard, 1936).

Apparently there was an interchange of customs between societies as with the Ibeji cult taken to Brazil by the Yorubas. Such individual customs would be very acceptable to the host community because they assisted in rationalizing their own fears of the portents of a twin-birth. With the passage of time and improved communications, the more severe sanctions have disappeared, but apprehension still probably remains as a legacy.

CHAPTER 2

Types of Twinning and Determination of Zygosity

G. CORNEY AND E. B. ROBSON

It is customary to refer to two types of twinning, namely *dizygotic* often
alternatively described as *dizygous, fraternal* or *binovular* and *monozygotic*
for which other descriptions include *monozygous, identical* or *uniovular;* however, these alternative names are best avoided on either biological or ety-
mological grounds (Edwards, 1968). For the purposes of this discussion we
will therefore use only the terms dizygotic (DZ) and monozygotic (MZ).

DIZYGOTIC TWINNING

Here two ova are released from the same or separate ovaries and each is
fertilised. In the normal menstrual cycle (Bulmer, 1970) several follicles begin
to ripen in each ovary, but only one of them develops into a mature Graafian
follicle destined to ovulate whilst the rest either stop growing or undergo
atresia. There is evidence for this in other species and the process is thought
to be controlled by a complex interplay of hormones which also probably
influence the relative follicular developments in the two ovaries. The situation
is mainly controlled by gonadotrophins and the recent use of these substances
in the treatment of infertility has increased our knowledge of follicular development and ovarian release substantially. For example, it has been possible to
examine (at laparoscopy) the ovaries of patients treated with such hormones
and it is thought that such therapy stimulates differentiation of many or all
of the available follicles into Graafian follicles. Using such techniques Edwards
and his co-workers (1973) found an average of five to six Graafian follicles in
each ovary irrespective of the amount of gonadotrophin administered. Twin
and other multiple pregnancies are, because of problems associated with
estimation of the dose and assessment of the response of an individual patient,

16

known to be a hazard of such treatment (Hack et al, 1970, 1972), thus providing 'therapeutic proof' for the association of gonadotrophins and multiple births, in particular those from more than one zygote, as such pregnancies have usually been multizygotic (Benirschke and Kim, 1973). An illustration of this is a case of twin pregnancy following the administration of gonadotrophins (Robertson and Grant, 1972) in which four corpora lutea were observed at operation for a ruptured tubal pregnancy; there were also many other stimulated but unruptured follicles. Similarly in a sextuplet pregnancy following gonadotrophin therapy it seemed at Caesarean section that a large number of follicles had ruptured (Lachelin et al, 1972).

There are, however, complexities involved in trying to associate ovarian morphology, for example the number of corpora lutea, with a twin pregnancy in order to determine the zygosity of the twins. Benirschke and Driscoll (1967) described a case of twin male embryos (found at total hysterectomy) with a monochorionic diamniotic placenta, but two corpora lutea were seen in the ovary also removed at operation. The authors presumed that either one ovum never became fertilised or implantation (of the second fertilised ovum) never took place. They cited a further case in which no trace of a corpus luteum could be found in the ovary (one having been previously removed) when monozygotic triplets were delivered by Caesarean section. On the other hand there is some evidence that two eggs can sometimes arise from one ovarian follicle (Corner, 1955; Strong and Corney, 1967) and multinucleate ova have been reported in man and other species (Kennedy and Donahue, 1969).

Thus there is evidence that twins can arise from two ova which after fertilisation become two zygotes; dizygotic twinning could therefore be described as a duplication of the normal process of conception. Monozygotic twinning in contrast is a gross deviation from the normal development of a single zygote. It is therefore hardly surprising that anomalies are more frequently associated with the latter process.

After fertilisation (Figure 2.1) the two zygotes pass down either the same or individual Fallopian tubes and implant on the wall of the uterus within the first week after conception. Such implantation might be on adjacent or remote parts of the uterine wall and this is probably a matter of chance. Since each of these zygotes can be regarded as a singleton pregnancy, development will proceed as for a normal conceptus with regard to placental differentiation and formation of the embryo and membranes. There will therefore be two placentae, each with a chorionic and amniotic membrane (Figure 2.1), but they may show various degrees of 'fusion' depending on the proximity of the implantation sites.

SUPERFECUNDATION AND SUPERFETATION

These phenomena imply that dizygotic twins might arise from more than one act of coitus either in a single menstrual cycle (superfecundation) or in different cycles (superfetation). Various reports are reviewed by Radasch (1921), Studdiford (1936), Deansley (1966) and Scrimgeour and Baker (1974).

Whilst there is evidence for superfecundation from blood group studies in

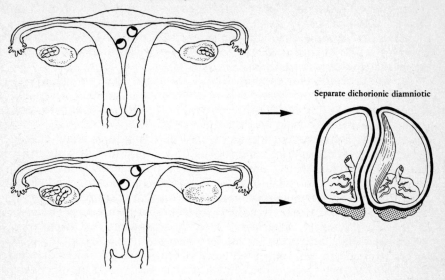

Two corpora lutea, two ova, separate implantation

Separate dichorionic diamniotic

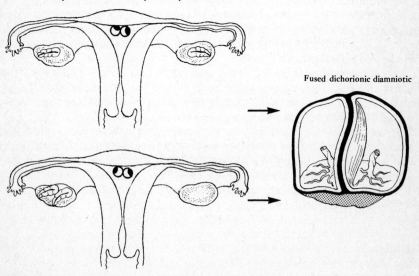

Two corpora lutea, two ova, adjacent implantation

Fused dichorionic diamniotic

Figure 2.1. Dizygotic twinning. The diagram demonstrates that the form of dichorionic placentation depends on the relative sites of implantation of the two zygotes. See text for explanation.

a single case (Gedda, 1951, 1961), demonstrating that twins had different fathers, other reports are less convincing, frequently being very old and describing differing degrees of pigmentation in the twins, often from hearsay evidence. Since the genetics of skin pigmentation are ill-understood it is difficult to accept such cases as conclusive evidence. Thus whilst superfecundation might occur in man it must be rare. Superfetation may be defined as the implantation of a second fertilised ovum in a uterus already containing a pregnancy of at least one month's duration and the subsequent simultaneous development of fetuses of different ages. Suppression of the inhibition of the corpus luteum of the initial pregnancy would be necessary for this state of affairs to exist and whilst this situation is theoretically possible, there is as yet no conclusive evidence that it does occur (Bulmer, 1970; Scrimgeour and Baker, 1974). Reports in the literature suggesting that it might, are mainly based on discrepancies in birth weight between the two babies. Substantial differences in birth weight are not uncommon amongst monochorionic pairs, due to intrauterine vascular competition and so, contrary to what might be expected, birth weight differences do not give unambiguous evidence in relation to time of conception. Therefore it remains to be proven whether superfetation does occur; at present it seems unlikely.

MONOZYGOTIC TWINNING

This is a gross aberration of normal development in which a single zygote divides to produce two embryos; it seems that this might happen at a variable time after fertilisation with consequent differing effects on the type of placentation and on the embryos. Useful general reviews of the process can be found in Corner (1955), Gedda (1951, 1961), Strong and Corney (1967), Benirschke and Driscoll (1967), Boyd and Hamilton (1970) and Bulmer (1970).

As Corner discusses in his 1955 paper, it was originally suspected that human monozygotic twinning might be a possibility from the fact that some pairs of human twins of similar appearance had a single placenta and were enclosed in a single (chorioamniotic) membrane. The existing morphological theory of single-ovum twinning has subsequently been built up on the basis of very few embryological specimens, but as Corner pointed out twenty years ago, this is in the main a paper theory which has been transferred into many established textbooks as proven. He emphasises (and twenty years on the situation does not seem to have changed much) that the whole theory behind the process should still be regarded very critically and whilst a useful classification (as for example the one he gives) can be used for discussion or teaching, one must not lose sight of the fact that the process is not one of stages but of continuous development in which various cells might themselves differ in their degree of differentiation. Benirschke and Kim (1973) also prefer to regard the time-scale as a 'continuum' and provide a useful diagram (Figure 2.2) which helps to stress the lack of rigid stages. The forms of placentation are shown diagrammatically in Figure 2.3.

When the zygote has first divided into two daughter cells or blastomeres, these cells may separate and still retain complete potentiality. Early work in support of this hypothesis is described by Hamilton (1954) and Boyd and Hamilton (1970), but more recently Moore (1973) discusses work on individual blastomeres of the rat, rabbit, mouse, pig and sheep, full potential having been shown to be present at the two to eight-cell stage of development in the mouse, rabbit and sheep. It is suggested that cellular specialisation does not take place until after the eight-cell stage of development and that all blastomeres of the earlier stages may be capable of full development into normal young.

Presuming therefore that this is possible in the case of human cells, each of the two blastomeres from the first division of a single zygote would become

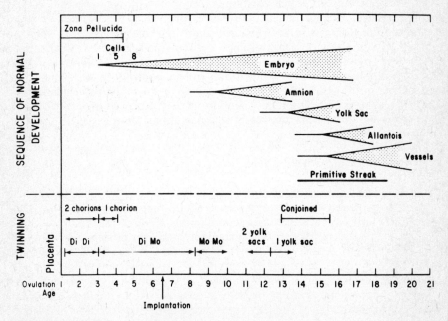

Figure 2.2. Diagram correlating the timing of embryological events and placentation in MZ twinning. Reprinted by permission from *New England Journal of Medicine* (1973), **288**, 1276 and Dr K. Benirschke.

a cell mass and both would pass down the Fallopian tube implanting either separately or together in the uterus. Thus the twins, although coming from a single zygote, would have individual placentae; in other words they would be dichorionic diamniotic. Early specimens of this type of monozygotic twinning have not been seen; Boyd and Hamilton (1970) describe a pair of dichorionic twin embryos of like sex, but it was presumably not possible to make an assessment of the zygosity. Thus there is, to use Corner's words, still only a 'paper version' of the origin of this type of twinning. However, there is evidence from other species that it might happen and studies of placentation and zygosity (as will be described in Chapter 3) in human twin pregnancies have shown that a small proportion of twins with dichorionic placentation are alike for sex and all genetic markers tested and are therefore

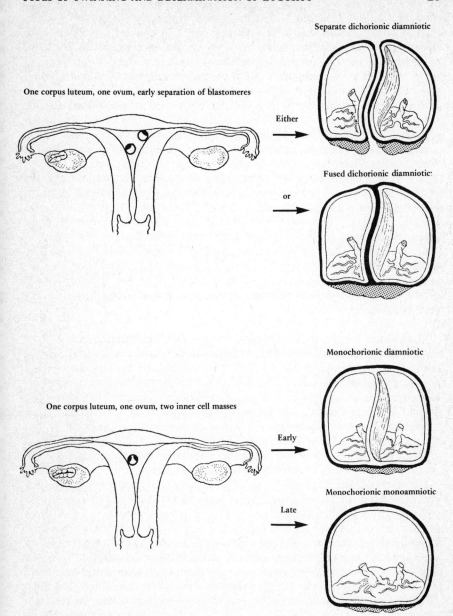

Figure 2.3. Monozygotic twinning. In the case of early separation of the blastomeres the form of dichorionic placentation depends on the relative sites of implantation of the two zygotes, as with dizygotic twinning (see Figure 2.1). Division at a later stage produces monochorionic placentation which can be either diamniotic or monoamniotic depending on the time of division.

probably monozygotic, but direct supporting evidence is lacking. This could theoretically be obtained from the observation of a single corpus luteum when dichorionic twins were delivered, but since, as has been described, this type of observation is open to misinterpretation, it is hard to see how the case can be 'proved'. However, it is clear that if this rationale for early MZ twinning is accepted, then conclusions about zygosity cannot be drawn from inspection of dichorionic diamniotic twin placentae, since their origin in terms of cell masses and subsequent transmission and implantation are essentially similar (Figures 2.1 and 2.3). The only difference might be that, since cell masses from a single zygote will presumably never pass down different Fallopian tubes, whereas those from two zygotes (if they came from different ovaries) might—thus if transmission along the same tube means closer implantation on the uterine wall (and it is not known if this is the case), then MZ twins might be expected to have fused dichorionic placentae more often than DZ twins. In fact, according to Bulmer (1970), this does not seem to be so, but there are several weaknesses in this argument such as the somewhat uncertain criteria on examination for 'fusion' and 'separation' of such placentae and also ignorance of the factors which control transmission in the Fallopian tube and subsequent implantation. It is not therefore clear how much inference can be drawn from data of this type as will be discussed in more detail in the next chapter.

If, however, twinning does not take place at such an early stage, division of the single cell mass will continue. This produces a ball of cells containing a cavity at one pole of which cells eventually destined to become the embryo are becoming isolated as the 'inner cell mass'. This area of enormous potential is recognisable about the fourth day and implantation occurs about the seventh day. At this stage the chorionic membrane is already established and therefore if twinning happens subsequently it will affect the inner cell mass only; thus it would be expected that there would be two amniotic cavities each containing an embryo, but only a single chorionic membrane and placental disc. The twins would therefore be monochorionic diamniotic.

Early monochorionic embryological specimens have been seen and a review and discussion of the various samples is given by Corner (1955) and Boyd and Hamilton (1970). There are very few such cases and they are of great interest, but in fact they actually represent a tiny series of extremely premature twin deliveries and as such only give information about early stages of development once this form of placentation has been established. They are not however necessarily informative about their *origin* and in any case there is no report of an embryo younger than two weeks estimated age. The most valuable information would be obtained from specimens within the first two weeks.

At about the end of the second week, the primitive streak is forming and even at this late stage twinning might occur if two embryonic nodules appear instead of one (Corner, 1955); in such a case there will only be a single amniotic cavity. Corner described a few embryos of this type, namely enclosed in a single amniotic cavity, the youngest being 24 days. He commented however that they were mostly in a poor state of preservation; two of them were pairs of conjoined twins (see below) providing supporting evidence for the theory that the twinning process can still happen after the amniotic membrane has been formed. An earlier (18 to 19-day) specimen with a single amniotic cavity, reported by Hertig (1967), also showed a conjoined germ disc. Twins formed at this point will therefore have monochorionic monoamniotic placentation; in other words, the same placenta and membrane structure as is found in a singleton pregnancy.

It has occasionally been suggested that in this (monoamniotic) type of twin placentation the cavity might initially have been double, but the dividing layers of amniotic membrane later fused and disappeared. This mechanism has been observed in other species, but there has never been convincing evidence from human twin placentae for the existence of such an amniotic septum earlier in development. It might therefore reasonably be concluded that if it happens at all in man it must be very rare (Corner, 1955; Benirschke and Driscoll, 1967).

CONJOINED TWINS

The latest stage at which twinning might occur, and perhaps better regarded as 'incomplete' twinning, results in a further subdivision of the monoamniotic group. If twinning takes place at the end of the second week of development, the amniotic membrane will have formed and the twins will be in the same amniotic cavity, but should this process be incomplete, then the twin embryos might not separate. The resulting pair are usually referred to as *conjoined twins* and a review of this phenomenon and various associated factors can be found in the monographs of Gedda (1961) and Bergsma (1967). The mechanism is not clear, but current thought is in favour of imperfect division of cellular elements in the germ disc. The alternative explanation (Szendi, 1939; Aird, 1959) that there might have been fusion of two cell masses has not received much support. It is difficult to know how this could be demonstrated in monozygotic twin embryos and in the case of dizygotic fusion one would also have to postulate fusion and disappearance of the dividing membranes, an exceedingly rare event in man as previously discussed. In addition conjoined twins are always of the same sex and there has not been a report of genetic differences between such twins; chromosome studies have been carried out in a few cases and the karyotypes have always been normal (Benirschke and Kim, 1973). Apparent phenotypic difference in sex is likely to be due to some form of hermaphroditism (Szendi, 1939; Khanna, Roy and Bhatt, 1969).

The theoretical origin of this group derives from even more speculation than for the other types of twinning previously described, as understandably embryological specimens are exceedingly rare. The cases described by Corner (1955) have already been mentioned and the same author reports another specimen (at about 10 weeks) in which the twins are separate but there was only a single umbilical cord. Ysander (1924, 1925), reviewing a number of cases of thoracopagus twins (united at the level of the thorax) described four such embryos, the youngest of which was thought to be about six weeks gestation. It is likely (Zimmermann, 1967) that many conjoined pairs are aborted early in development and that the few cases seen at term are not representative of the true incidence. The same author also points out that, although the assumption is usually made that such twins originate by incomplete fission of the inner cell mass, the possibility cannot be excluded that such partial splitting could have happened before the blastocyst implanted in the endometrium. This would be in keeping with the theme discussed earlier with regard to 'normal' twins that we know very little about the timing of events within the inner cell mass. It is said that differentiation of the germ-disc has taken place before the late stage at which division would produce either monoamniotic (normal) twins or conjoined twins and one might therefore expect to find the greatest degrees of dissimilarity such as 'lateral asymmetry' (mirror imaging) in such pairs (Benirschke and Driscoll, 1967). Others state that this phenomenon does not occur amongst MZ twins in general more often than would be expected by chance (Bulmer, 1970) and opinion is also divided about lateral asymmetry in conjoined twins (Walker, 1952; Nance, 1959); in any case the hypothesis is open to criticism from the point of view of lack of precise knowledge about timing and differentiation as has just been discussed. A further complication about suppositions with regard to the timing of the conjoined twinning process can be found in the occasional descriptions of triplet and even quadruplet pregnancies in which such pairs were delivered with a normal infant (Rudolph, Michaels and Nichols, 1967; Tan et al, 1971b; Vestergaard, 1972). On present reasoning this suggests that (in the case of triplets) there might have been an additional early twinning event, as in one of the triplet sets one of the infants had a separate placenta, whereas the conjoined twins presumably arose some days later in the first two weeks or so after fertilisation (Benirschke and Kim, 1973).

There is substantial variation both in the morphology of the umbilical cords in such pairs, as they may be forked or fused (Benirschke and Driscoll, 1967) and in the number of cord vessels which might vary from two to seven (Rudolph, Michaels and Nichols, 1967; Nichols, Blattner and Rudolph, 1967).

The frequency of conjoined twins in reports in the literature is somewhat variable (Rudolph, Michaels and Nichols, 1967; Beischer and Fortune, 1968; Tan et al, 1971a); an estimate for England and Wales has been made from national data by Bulmer (1970) and this particular frequency seems to be rather more than one in 100 000 births or one in 400 monozygotic twin maternities. The suggestion that conjoined twins might be commoner in Africa, in particular in Nigeria (Aird, 1954, 1959) is not supported by recent prospective studies there in which only one such pair was found amongst over 3000 twin births (Nylander, 1974). It seems likely (Rudolph, Michaels and Nichols, 1967) that the frequency probably does not differ between countries and this is not really surprising as it is likely that conjoined twins always arise from one zygote and there is no racial variation in monozygotic twinning throughout the world (Bulmer, 1970; Nylander, 1971b).

There is a strange anomaly in the sex distribution amongst conjoined twins in that about 70 per cent are female (Rudolph, Michaels and Nichols, 1967; Benirschke and Kim, 1973) and the reason for this is not known.

The cause of such a gross aberration of the normal process of development in humans is not known but is has been shown with trout (Stockard, 1921) and zebra fish (Ingalls, Philbrook and Majima, 1969) that hypoxia and alterations in temperature of the water are associated with the subsequent appearance of conjoined twins. They have also been produced following experimental delay in fertilisation in the frog (Witschi, 1970) and after tera- togens have been given to hamsters (Ferm, 1969) and it is suggested (Ingalls and Bazemore, 1969) that prenatal environmental disturbances or agents of this nature might be responsible for human conjoined twinning.

Such experimental evidence is presumably also applicable to the causation of monozygotic twinning in general, as it seems not unreasonable to assume that there might be common factors in the production of deviations in the developmental pattern of a single zygote.

HETEROKARYOTIC MONOZYGOTIC TWINS

In recent years a number of pairs of twins thought likely to be monozygotic either from study of blood groups and other genetic markers or from mono- chorionic placentation, have been found to be discordant for chromosome anomalies. The first such case, described by Turpin et al (1961), was in a pair of twins of different sex, the female showing the clinical picture of Turner's syndrome and on chromosome study they were found to be respectively XY and XO. However, blood group studies gave a high probability that they were monozygotic twins. It was therefore presumed that they had been derived from an XY zygote with the loss of one of the Y chromosomes. Subsequently other pairs, presumed to be monozygotic, have been found to be discordant for Turner's syndrome and also for mongolism. The subject has been reviewed by Nielsen (1967) and Benirschke (Benirschke and Driscoll, 1967; Benirschke, 1972b; Benirschke and Kim, 1973). Further cases are those described by Kerr and Rashad (1966) involving discordance for trisomy of a group C chromo- some and more recently for trisomy G and acardia (Scott and Ferguson- Smith, 1973).

It is thought that after mitotic division the chromatids are not evenly distributed and that this error takes place at about the same time as the twinning event (post-zygotic non-disjunction). Most of the cases are thought to have had monochorionic placentae which, whilst providing strong evidence for monozygosity, also means that there will almost certainly have been some mixture of blood elements through vascular communications in the placenta. Therefore fetal chromosome findings from blood (lymphocyte) culture are likely to be at variance with those from tissue (fibroblast) culture. An addi- tional complication is that if twinning and non-disjunction happen after the chorion has been established (monochorionic placentation), the chromosomal composition of the chorionic tissue will presumably be different from that of the fetus and also from the amnion (in the case of *monochorionic diamniotic* placentation). Such studies (culture of the placental membranes) have not been carried out, but they would be of great interest if such an opportunity ever presented. One might then find evidence of placento-fetal mosaicism, the consequences of which are unknown (Benirschke and Driscoll, 1967). This hypothetical situation is a further reason for retaining the placenta for special study after a twin birth because even if for example tissue culture studies are not possible, accurate recording of details of the type of placentation (dichorionic or monochorionic) would give some guidance as to the timing of the twinning event with the proviso already discussed that placental membrane relationships are only a guide and may not necessarily give an accurate index of the stage at which differentiation of the two *embryos* began to differ (Corner, 1955).

If this mainly hypothetical (though to some extent substantiated by embryological specimens) chronological programme for monozygotic twinning during the first two weeks after fertilisation is accepted, it can be seen that there are (at least) three different varieties of MZ twins, namely dichorionic diamniotic, monochorionic diamniotic and monochorionic monoamniotic.

THIRD TYPE OF TWINS

It has occasionally been postulated (Mijsberg, 1957; Nance, 1959) that in addition to these two forms of twinning, there might be a 'third' type. This suggestion was discussed by Danforth in 1916, but presumably in part due to difficulties of investigating the hypothesis, it seems not to have been studied in any detail for many years. There are several theoretical ways in which this might happen, but central to all the mechanisms is the fact that the ovum is fertilised by two sperms. The resulting pair of twins would thus neither be dizygotic (two ova + two sperms) nor monozygotic (one ovum + one sperm), but rather an amalgam of these two possibilities, the maternal contribution of genes being the same for both members of the pair and any genetic differences between them being attributable to the father. The possible mechanisms for this hypothetical third type of twinning have been discussed by Mijsberg (1957) and Bulmer (1970) and the requisite stages in the maturation of the ovum have been observed in other species. The result of the fertilisation of one ovum by two sperms (dispermy) to produce a mosaic singleton has been demonstrated in man several times (Race and Sanger, 1975), but it still remains to be proven whether a similar mechanism could result in more than one individual.

In order to prove if a third type of twinning does exist, it has been suggested that genetic markers from DZ twins should be studied in order to see whether they are similar (concordant) more often than would be expected by chance amongst DZ pairs. Reviewing data for the MN and ABO blood group systems amongst twins which had been published by Schiff and von Verschuer over twenty years earlier, Mijsberg (1957) did find such concordance and therefore support for the hypothesis for the existence of a third type of twin pair. However, this was not the case when the same author examined data for the P blood group. Matsunaga (1966) also studied the

ABO and MN blood group systems and did not find any evidence for the existence of such pairs. Bulmer (1970) has made a comprehensive review of the whole problem including analysis of blood group concordance in 1848 pairs of twins, some of which are drawn from the data studied earlier by Mijsberg. Bulmer found good agreement between the observed and expected proportions of twins who are concordant for the markers tested. From this result and from further analyses of blood group data and the frequency of concordance for mongolism amongst DZ twins, Bulmer concludes that there is no evidence to support the existence of a third form of twinning and that if such pairs do exist they must be very rare.

Thus it can be concluded that (with possible rare exceptions) all non-identical twins are dizygotic.

DETERMINATION OF ZYGOSITY

The origins of the two types of twins from one and two zygotes respectively means that monozygotic (MZ) twins must be alike for all their genetically determined characteristics, whereas dizygotic (DZ) twins are no more alike genetically than any pair of siblings. It follows immediately that a single difference between the members of a twin pair proves their DZ nature, whereas the absence of a detectable difference is not absolute evidence of monozygosity, but becomes more and more indicative the more exhaustive the investigation.

Genetically determined characters which are the most useful for zygosity testing are those which show commonly occurring variation, have a simple mode of inheritance and are relatively unaffected by the environment. The red cell antigens (commonly referred to as the blood groups, although there are now many more 'groups' detectable in blood by biochemical rather than by serological techniques) were the first such characters to be widely used in testing twins. More recently the discovery of widespread variation in the structure of serum proteins and red cell enzymes, detectable by electrophoresis, has increased the number of informative systems. Developments in histocompatibility testing have also provided genetically determined markers on the white cells. More and more such marker systems are being discovered, and provided that the genetical basis is clearly understood, any such system can be incorporated into zygosity testing. Which systems are in fact utilised depends upon several factors, including the availability of biological samples, the expertise required for any particular test and the cost and availability of reagents. Considering especially the problem in the newborn, tests which can be performed on a sample of cord blood are the easiest to arrange. The most informative red cell antigens, *ABO*, *Rh*, and *MNSs*, can be determined by any blood bank, but the red cell enzyme and serum protein typing is performed in a more limited number of centres, usually those specialising in biochemical genetics. Most of the systems are, however, fairly robust, and samples can be sent by post without elaborate precautions. Histocompatibility testing, at least for the *HL-A* locus, is generally available in each major hospital area, but here the timing is more critical. Additional information is obtainable in the case of the newborn since placental tissue is generally available. Some genetically determined enzyme variations cannot be detected in red cells, but can be determined in other tissues. Some are found in most solid tissues, whilst one at least, placental alkaline phosphatase, is restricted to the placenta. It has been shown that the enzyme characteristics of the placenta are determined solely by the fetal genotype, so the tissue constitution of the newborn can be determined in this way. Only a small piece of tissue is required for biochemical testing, about 10 g is sufficient, and this can be kept frozen, without fixing, until it can be tested.

Such clearly defined genetically determined systems are undoubtedly the most objective way in which to determine zygosity, and with their ever increasing number and availability have largely displaced older methods which were based on morphological similarity. It is a matter of common experience that the morphological method works most of the time, for bigger children and adults, since MZ twins are often difficult to tell apart, but this observation is difficult to quantify since the genetical components of size, shape and pigmentation are not simple to interpret. In the newborn situation this approach is clearly unproductive. Not only are most morphological characters undeveloped but those that are present, such as weight, still show pronounced maternal effects, some genetical and some environmental. Indeed some MZ twin pairs, such as those suffering from the twin-transfusion syndrome, may show more dramatic size differences than DZ twins. However, some quantifiable morphological characteristics have been used fairly extensively in the past, in particular finger and palm prints. These characters are fully developed at birth and can be obtained from babies, though not without considerable difficulty! The total finger ridge count, and the size of the angle subtended by certain lines on the palm are two measures which can be used to give a relative probability of zygosity.

So far we have considered the qualitative and quantitative characters which may be utilised in determining the zygosity of *any* newborn twin pair. Occasionally, of course, critical evidence regarding zygosity may be derived for a particular pair from the occurrence of a rare event. If one of the twins suffers from a rare genetically determined disease, such as phenylketonuria, whilst the other does not, then this is clear evidence of dizygosity. If they are alike for such a rare genetic anomaly, then the probability of their being dizygotic is reduced in an exactly definable way, as will be outlined in a following section. In the subsequent procedures described for the determination of zygosity, such rare events will be ignored.

The process of zygosity determination proceeds by elimination. Dizygosity can definitely be established for those pairs differing in sex or in any of the red cell or serum protein systems. There are, of course, very rare exceptions to this claim, as in the case of those phenotypically male–female pairs who are chromosomally XY and XO, and probably derived from only one XY zygote where one twin has lost the Y chromosome at an early cell division. Similar exceptions in the serological and biochemical systems are theoretically possible, due to the loss or inactivation of a particular gene locus, but no case has so far been described. Diagnoses depending upon only *one* difference are, of course, worrying, although they must be expected to occur, especially when the full range of tests is not carried out. In practical terms it is advisable to repeat the critical test, preferably on a fresh blood sample, to reduce the possibility of technical error.

The pairs who are alike for all markers constitute both the truly MZ pairs and also the DZ pairs who by chance do not happen to differ in the systems investigated. The relative chance of dizygosity obviously gets less the more information is available and methods to quantify this probability form the topic of the rest of this section.

The calculation is most straightforward where the parents are also tested, as the problem can then be exactly defined. On the hypothesis of the dizygotic origin the genotypes of the twins are subject to the laws determining the genotypes of *any* two children of the same parents, so that if we take twin 1 as given, and have information about the parents, then we can usually calculate exactly the probability that twin 2 will have the same markers as twin 1.

It is necessary at this point to explain in a general way the mode of inheritance of the systems used, and to define a few additional terms. The observed individual characteristic, be it the result of a serological reaction or a biochemical test, is described as the *phenotype*, whilst the underlying genetical constitution is known as the *genotype*. The phenotype may fully define the genotype as in the AB type in the red cell antigen system *ABO*. Each individual has two alleles (or genes) at a particular locus, one derived from the mother and one from the father, and since an AB individual shows both A and B characteristics serologically, his two alleles are fully described. However, an A type individual shows only one specificity and we cannot know from the serological test whether his genotype is *AA* or *AO*, for the O allele is not detected in the test. The doubt is sometimes resolved by family studies since an A individual with an O spouse can have O children if he is *AO*, but only A children if he is *AA*. Fortunately such complications are confined to the red cell antigens, and in the enzyme and protein systems detected biochemically both gene products are directly observable, and so the phenotype completely defines the genotype.

Having made what deductions are possible regarding the genotypes of all family members we can proceed to estimate the probability that truly DZ twins would be alike for the markers tested. Consider the Gc (group-specific component) system. There are two alleles Gc^1 and Gc^2, such that Gc^1Gc^1

Table 2.1. *Segregation of phenotypes in the offspring of possible mating types, for a system having two alleles.*

		Phenotype of offspring		
Mating type		1	2-1	2
(a)	1 × 1	1.0	0	0
(b)	1 × 2-1	0.5	0.5	0
(c)	1 × 2	0	1.0	0
(d)	2-1 × 2-1	0.25	0.5	0.25
(e)	2-1 × 2	0	0.5	0.5
(f)	2 × 2	0	0	1.0

individuals are phenotypically 1, Gc^2Gc^1 individuals type 2-1 and Gc^2Gc^2 individuals type 2. Table 2.1 shows the array of mating types which are possible and the segregation of phenotypes within those families. Mating types a, c and f are uninformative in zygosity determination since the children cannot differ in genotype. Mating types, b, d and e are informative since more than one type of child is possible. Consider the mating type 1 × 2-1 (b), where the observed twin pair is of type 2-1. We ask the question: given that twin 1 is of type 2-1, what is the probability that twin 2 is also of type 2-1? We see from Table 2.1 that the probability of a child in that family being of type 2-1 is 0.5, that is, it could equally likely be type 1 or type 2-1. By multiplying together such probabilities for each system we obtain the combined probability that twin 2 will be genetically identical to twin 1. It is impossible here to go into greater detail regarding the genetics of the individual systems, but these can be found in Race and Sanger's *Blood Groups in Man* and Giblett's *Genetic Markers in Human Blood*. Whilst the basic principle for its use in zygosity determination is the same, each system has its own complexities which should be borne in mind. In testing the newborn, for instance, it is necessary to remember that the red cell antigens P and Lewis are unreliable. The probabilities for all the enzyme and serum protein markers can easily be calculated from first principles, as described for the *Gc* system, but the problem is more complicated in the case of some of the blood groups where the phenotype does not fully define the genotype. In these cases it is necessary to enumerate all the possible mating types which could produce children of the given type, and weight the probabilities by the relative frequency with which these matings occur in the population. This requires additional information on gene frequencies, and is also tedious and repetitious, and so Race and Sanger have provided tables for the most commonly occurring situations in several of the blood group systems (Table 2.2).

Table 2.2. *Relative chances in favour of dizygosity of twin pairs; parental phenotypes known but genotype of at least one parent unknown. Some useful examples for Northern Europeans.*

Mating	Twins both	Relative chance of dizygosity	Mating	Twins both	Relative chance of dizygosity
$A_1 \times O$	A_1	0.6113	Fy(a+) × Fy(a+)	Fy(a+)	0.8815
$A_2 \times O$	A_2	0.5474	Fy(a+) × Fy(a−)	Fy(a+)	0.7072
B × O	B	0.5424			
$A_1 \times A_1$	A_1	0.8224	Jk(a+) × Jk(a+)	Jk(a+)	0.9102
$A_1 \times A_2$	A_1	0.6113	Jk(a+) × Jk(a−)	Jk(a+)	0.7571
$A_1 \times A_2$	A_2	0.3122			
			Do(a+) × Do(a+)	Do(a+)	0.8831
$P_1 \times P_1$	P_1	0.9034	Do(a+) × Do(a−)	Do(a+)	0.7100
$P_1 \times P_2$	P_1	0.7700			
			Xg(a−) × Xg(a+)	Xg(a+)	0.8303
			father mother		
Le(a−) × Le(a−)	Le(a−)⎫		Xg(a+) × Xg(a+)	Xg(a+)	0.8303
sec. sec.	sec. ⎬ 0.9123		father mother	sons	
Le(a+) × Le(a−)	Le(a−)⎭				
non-sec. sec.	sec. ⎫ 0.7634				

From Race and Sanger (1975), with permission of the authors and Blackwell Scientific Publications.

Table 2.3. *A comparison of zygosity determination in a particular family, with and without parental data.*

	Phenotype of			Using parental data		Ignoring parental data	
System	Father	Mother	Twins	Chance of DZ twins in this family having these phenotypes	Chance of MZ twins in this family having these phenotypes	Chance of DZ twins	Chance of MZ twins
ABO	B	O	O	0.50	1.00	0.6891	1.00
MNSs	NN	MN	MN	0.50	1.00	0.6246	1.00
Rh	R_1R_2	R_1r	R_2r	0.25	1.00	0.4179	1.00
Kell	K−	K−	K−	1.00	1.00	0.9548	1.00
Duffy	Fy(a+)	Fy(a−)	Fy(a−)	0.50	1.00	0.6235	1.00
ADA	1	1	1	1.00	1.00	0.9409	1.00
GPT	2-1	2-1	2-1	0.50	1.00	0.6250	1.00
ES-D	2-1	2-1	2-1	0.50	1.00	0.5438	1.00
Gc	2-1	1	1	0.50	1.00	0.7569	1.00
Pi	M	MS	MS	0.50	1.00	0.5215	1.00
Sex			Male	0.50	1.00	0.5000	1.00
Initial chance				0.70	0.30	0.7000	0.30
Combined chance after testing				0.0007	0.30	0.0048	0.30

The probability that these twins are monozygotic is 0.30/0.3007 = 0.9976.

If the parental data had not been available the probability would have been 0.30/0.3048 = 0.9842.

Adapted from Race and Sanger, *Blood Groups in Man*, 6th edition. The family was tested by the MRC Human Biochemical Genetics Unit, University College London, and was investigated clinically by Dr. R. H. Lindenbaum of the MRC Population Genetics Unit, Oxford.

A worked example of zygosity determination where both parents have been tested is given in Table 2.3. The various probabilities on the alternative hypotheses of mono- and dizygosity are listed for all the systems tested. In the case of the ABO groups the fact that the B father had O children indicates that his genotype is *BO* and not *BB*. If the children had been of type B then the father's genotype would have been uncertain and it would have been necessary to use the probability value listed in Table 2.2 for this mating type. Similarly the segregation of the *Duffy* phenotypes in the children defines the father's genotype. *PGM*$_1$ and *AK* have had to be omitted from this calculation since they are not inherited independently of *Rh* and *ABO* which have been used. This restriction, due to genetical linkage, is described more fully in the legend to Table 2.9. In addition to the markers, the fact that the twins are of the same sex allows one to reduce the probability of dizygosity by a further factor of O.5. A further factor, described as the Initial Chance, is not specific for any particular family, but utilises the observation from British population data that the overall rates of DZ and MZ twinning are roughly in the proportion of 7:3, so that before any investigation at all is attempted the twins are 2.3 times more likely to be DZ than MZ. For other populations different rates of DZ and MZ twinning may need to be used. All these individual probabilities are multiplied together to give a final combined probability on

Table 2.4. *Relative chances in favour of dizygotic twin pairs in a system of two alleles.*

Genotypic		Phenotypic	
Twin pair both	Relative chance in favour of dizygotic twins	Twin pair both	Relative chance in favour of dizygotic twins ·
AA	$\frac{1}{4}(1 + p)^2$	$\tilde{A}$	$1 - \frac{1}{4}q^2(3 + q)/(1 + q)$
Aa	$\frac{1}{2}(1 + pq)$		
aa	$\frac{1}{4}(1 + q)^2$	ã	$\frac{1}{4}(1 + q)^2$

From Smith and Penrose (1955), with permission of the former author, the editor of *Annals of Human Genetics* and Cambridge University Press.

Table 2.5. *Relative chances of dizygotic twin pairs when the ABO blood groups are the same.*

Twin pair both	Relative chance of dizygotic twins
O	0.6891
A_1 $\Big\}$ A A_2	0.6470 $\Big\}$ 0.6945 0.4824
B	0.4741
A_1B $\Big\}$ AB A_2B	0.3239 $\Big\}$ 0.3435 0.2849

From Smith and Penrose (1955)—see footnote to Table 2.4.

each hypothesis. In the family described the probability that the twins are MZ is 0.9976. We should only be mistaken in our diagnosis once in 250 times. This family is by no means exceptional, and indeed was not exhaustively investigated since neither the placenta nor white cells were available for testing.

Where the parents are not tested the exact probability cannot be calculated, but an estimate can be arrived at based on the gene frequency in the general population and assuming random mating. The general formulae for calculating the probabilities of dizygosity in two-allele systems are given in Table 2.4 and the formulae can be extended for use in multi-allelic systems. Smith and Penrose (1955) have calculated values for these probabilities for the *ABO*, *Rh* and *MNSs* systems and these are reproduced in Tables 2.5, 2.6 and 2.7. Race and Sanger's calculations for the other blood groups are given in Table 2.8. Values for the red cell and tissue enzyme systems and serum proteins are given in Table 2.9 together with some notes on the criteria determining their inclusion, and some restrictions on their use. All these tables are based on gene frequency estimates for Great Britain and are therefore not applicable in areas where the gene frequencies differ appreciably.

Table 2.6. *Relative chances in favour of dizygotic twin pairs when the Rhesus blood groups are the same.*

							Twin pair both	
							Phenotype	
							Reactions with anti-	Relative chance in favour of dizygotic pairs
$C + C^w$	c	D	E	C^w	e		Most likely genotype	
−	+	−	−	−	+		cde/cde rr	0.4821
−	+	+	−	−	+		cDe/cde R_0r	0.3684
−	+	−	+	−	+		cdE/cde $R''r$	0.3522
−	+	−	+	−	−		cdE/cdE $R''R''$	0.2500
−	+	+	+	−	−		cDE/cDE R_2R_2	0.3321
−	+	+	+	−	+		cDE/cde R_2r	0.4179
+	+	−	−	−	+		Cde/cde $R'r$	0.3512
+	+	+	−	−	+		CDe/cde R_1r	0.5400
+	+	+	−	+	+		C^wDe/cde R_1^wr	0.3599
+	+	−	+	−	+		cdE/Cde $R''R'$	0.2735
+	+	+	+	−	+		CDe/cDE R_1R_2	0.4241
+	+	+	+	−	−		cDE/CDE R_2R_z	0.2853
+	+	+	+	+	+		C^wDe/cDE $R_1^wR_2$	0.2943
+	−	−	−	−	+		Cde/Cde $R'R'$	0.2500
+	−	+	−	−	+		CDe/CDe R_1R_1	0.5021
+	−	+	−	+	+		C^wDe/CDe $R_1^wR_1$	0.3657
+	−	+	+	−	+		CDe/CDE R_1R_z	0.3546
+	−	+	+	+	−		CDE/CDE R_2R_z	0.2500
+	−	+	+	+	+		C^wDe/CDE $R_1^wR_z$	0.2500

From Smith and Penrose (1955)—see footnote to Table 2.4.

A worked example is given in Table 2.10. This does not refer to an observed twin pair, but an imaginary set where the most commonly occurring phenotype has been assumed at each locus, so that the combined probability of dizygosity is as high as it could possibly be for this set of markers. Such an individual, however, is quite unlikely to occur, despite his 'commonness' as most individuals are a mixture of common and less common types, thus making the probability of dizygosity lower. The vast majority of twin pairs could therefore be diagnosed as MZ with less than a one per cent level of error. A comparison is made in Table 2.3 of the efficiency of zygosity determination with and without knowledge of the parental genotypes. In this family there is a fourfold improvement in efficiency when the parental data are used. However, it should be remembered that this could easily be offset by adding information on the placental tissue phenotypes which is not included in the table because the genotypes of the parents for tissue-specific systems are generally unobtainable.

Table 2.7. *Relative chances in favour of dizygotic twin pairs when the MNSs blood groups are the same.*

Anti-M, -N, -S, -s sera available		Anti-M, -N, -S sera available	
Twin pair both	Relative chance in favour of dizygotic twins	Twin pair both	Relative chance in favour of dizygotic twins
MMSS	0.3888	MS	0.5161
MMSs	0.4176		
MMss	0.4116	*MsMs*	0.4116
MNSS	0.3417	MNS	0.5044
MNSs	0.4556		
MNss	0.4733	*MsNs*	0.4733
NNSS	0.2915	NS	0.4138
NNSs	0.3831		
NNss	0.4827	*NsNs*	0.4827

From Smith and Penrose (1955)—see footnote to Table 2.4.

It is often claimed that skin grafting is the only conclusive way of determining the zygosity of like-sexed twins. This has not been proposed here since the criteria adopted have included the ready availability of samples. Skin grafting is an elaborate procedure and certainly inappropriate in the newborn. The claim of its unique efficiency can also be questioned. The contention that skin grafts only 'take' between individuals of identical genotype is of course stating the case too dramatically. Only those loci which control rejection are relevant and their nature and number are not yet completely known, although they are clearly multiple and include the *ABO* locus and genes within the *MHC* (major histocompatibility) complex. What skin grafting does is to test for concordance at all these loci in one test, and is not, in principle, different from adding together the results from several different red cell antigen or enzyme markers which are determined separately. Whereas in the latter case the exact probability of monozygosity can be estimated when the twins are alike, in the case of skin grafting it cannot, since the genetics oɟ the process is incompletely understood. Since it has been shown that procedures which do not inconvenience the twins in any way give an error rate in diagnosis of less than one per cent at worst, the use of skin grafting would seem to be both unnecessary and unethical.

Further evidence relating to the problem of zygosity can be derived from finger and palm prints. Early investigations used the type of finger-tip patterns, but the more recently employed technique of ridge counting is preferable

Table 2.8. *Relative chances in favour of a dizygotic twin pair when the P, Lutheran, Kell, Secretor (or Lewis), Duffy, Kidd, Yt, Dombrock, Colton and Xg phenotypes are the same.*

System	Twin pair both	Relative chance in favour of dizygotic twins
P	P_1	0.8489
	P_2	0.5699
Lutheran	Lu(a+b−) ⎫ Lu(a+)	0.2699 ⎫
	Lu(a+b+) ⎬	0.5187 ⎬ 0.5337
	Lu(a−b+) Lu(a−)	0.9614 ⎭
Kell	K+k− ⎫ K+	0.2734 ⎫
	K+k+ ⎬	0.5218 ⎬ 0.5394
	K−k+ K−͗	0.9548 ⎭
Secretor	Non-secretor [Le(a+)]	0.5425
(or Lewis)	Secretor [Le(a−)]	0.8681
Duffy	Fy(a+b−) ⎫ Fy(a+)	0.5047 ⎫
	Fy(a+b+) ⎬	0.6219 ⎬ 0.8099
	Fy(a−b+) Fy(a−)	0.6235 ⎭
Kidd	Jk(a+b−) ⎫ Jk(a+)	0.5732 ⎫
	Jk(a+b+) ⎬	0.6249 ⎬ 0.8616
	Jk(a−b+) Jk(a−)	0.5519 ⎭
Yt	Yt(a+b−) Yt(b−)	0.9591
	Yt(a+b+) ⎫ Yt(b+)	0.5198 ⎫
	Yt(a−b+) ⎬	0.2711 ⎬ 0.5356
Dombrock	Do(a+b−) ⎫ Do(a+)	0.5041 ⎫
	Do(a+b+) ⎬	0.6218 ⎬ 0.8094
	Do(a−b+) Do(a−)	0.6241 ⎭
Colton	Co(a+b−) Co(b−)	0.9604
	Co(a+b+) ⎫ Co(b+)	0.5192 ⎫
	Co(a−b+) ⎬	0.2504 ⎬ 0.5345
Xg	male Xg(a+)	0.8310
	male Xg(a−)	0.6690
	female Xg(a+)	0.9573
	female Xg(a−)	0.6690

From Race and Sanger (1975)—see footnote to Table 2.2.

Table 2.9. *Relative chances in favour of dizygosity for a twin pair alike for a given genetically determined character. Values for 11 systems useful in Great Britain when testing the newborn. Based on data in the records of the MRC Human Biochemical Genetics Unit, University College London.*

Enzyme or serum protein system	Twin pair of like phenotype	Relative chance in favour of dizygosity
Tissue enzymes typed on placenta		
Placental alkaline phosphatase	1	0.7006
Pl	2-1	0.5606
	2	0.3856
	3-1	0.4678
	3	0.2938
	3-2	0.3417
Phosphoglucomutase, locus 3	1	0.7569
PGM_3	2-1	0.5962
	2	0.3969
Red cell enzymes		
Acid phosphatase, locus 1	A	0.4624
ACP_1	BA	0.5937
	B	0.6320
	CA	0.3615
	CB	0.4248
	C	0.2756
Phosphoglucomutase, locus 1	1	0.7788
PGM_1	2-1	0.5899
	2	0.3813
Adenylate kinase	1	0.9555
AK	2-1	0.5215
	2	0.2730
Adenosine deaminase	1	0.9409
ADA	2-1	0.5282
	2	0.2809
Esterase-D	1	0.9054
ES-D	2-1	0.5438
	2	0.3008
Glutamic-pyruvic transaminase	1	0.5646
GPT	2-1	0.6250
	2	0.5588
Serum proteins		
Group-specific component	1	0.7569
Gc	2-1	0.5962
	2	0.3969
α_1-antitrypsin	M	0.9555
Pi *S or other non-M types	MS*	0.5215
	S*	0.2730
Haptoglobin (sometimes developed	1-1	0.4761
Hp in the newborn)	2-1	0.6178
	2-2	0.6561

Notes for Table 2.9

CRITERIA FOR INCLUSION:

(a) The system must be adequately developed in the newborn.
(b) There must be no confusion with a maternal contribution, as in the *Gm* system in serum.
(c) Samples for testing should be readily available, i.e., cord blood and a small piece of placenta.
(d) The gene frequencies should be such that the amount of laboratory work required is not disproportionate to the information derived regarding zygosity. A frequency of about 0.95 for the most common allele has been selected as the limit of usefulness, as higher than this the factor contributed to the calculation of zygosity by the most common phenotype is greater than 0.95.

SOME RESTRICTIONS ON USING ALL THE SYSTEMS TESTED: Linked genes (i.e., genes at loci fairly close to each other on the same chromosome) are not inherited independently and so both systems cannot be used in the calculation of zygosity. This applies to the linked pairs *Rh* and *PGM$_1$*, *AK* and *ABO*, and *Lu* and *Se*, as far as is known at present (December 1974). It is therefore economical in testing to omit *PGM$_1$*, *AK* and *Se* typing, especially since the information regarding the blood groups is of value in itself.

Table 2.10. *An example of the use of the blood group tables (2.5, 2.6, 2.7, 2.8) and Table 2.9 in determining the chance of dizygosity in a twin pair alike for all blood group and biochemical markers and of the most common phenotype at all loci.*

Marker system	Phenotype	Relative chance of dizygosity for a particular system	Relative chance of monozygosity for a particular system
Initial odds		0.7000	0.3
Sex	Female	0.5000	1.0
ABO	A	0.6945	1.0
MNSs	MS	0.5161	1.0
Rh	R$_1$r	0.5400	1.0
Kell	K−	0.9548	1.0
Secretor	Sec	0.8681	1.0
Duffy	Fy(a+)	0.8099	1.0
Kidd	Jk(a+)	0.8616	1.0
Dombrock	Do(a+)	0.8094	1.0
Xg	Xg(a+)	0.9573	1.0
Pl	1	0.7006	1.0
PGM$_3$	1	0.7569	1.0
ACP$_1$	B	0.6320	1.0
ADA	1	0.9409	1.0
ES-D	1	0.9054	1.0
GPT	2-1	0.6250	1.0
Gc	1	0.7569	1.0
Pi	M	0.9555	1.0
Combined chance after testing		0.0056	0.3

Chance of dizygosity = 0.0056/0.3056 = 0.0183

P, Yt and *Hp* have not been used as they are not fully developed in the newborn, and *Lu, PGM$_1$* and *AK* because they are linked to *Sec, Rh* and *ABO* respectively.

Table 2.11. *Relative chances in favour of dizygotic twin pairs according to differences in total finger ridge count.*

Difference in total count	Percentage of pairs Monozygotic twins (m)	Like-sexed sibs (d)	Relative chance in favour of a dizygotic pair (d/m)
0-2	7.69	3.96	} 0.23
3-7	26.92	3.96	
8-12	26.92	6.93	0.26
13-17	19.23	6.93	0.36
18-22	7.69	5.94	0.77
23-27	5.77	5.94	1.03
28-32	3.85	4.95	1.29
33-37	0.00	5.94	} 33.97
38-	1.92	55.45	
Total	99.99	100.00	1.00

From Smith and Penrose (1955)—see footnote to Table 2.4.

Table 2.12. *Relative chances in favour of dizygotic twin pairs according to differences in the sum of the left and right maximal atd palmar angles.*

Differences (degrees)	Percentage of pairs Monozygotic twins (m)	Sibs (d)	Relative chance in favour of a dizygotic pair (d/m)
0	5.00	2.90	0.59
1-2	17.50	8.71	0.50
3-5	26.25	16.77	0.66
6-9	25.00	20.00	0.80
10-19	20.00	27.10	1.36
20-	6.25	24.52	3.92
Total	100.00	100.00	1.00

From Smith and Penrose (1955)—see footnote to Table 2.4.

as it enables the pattern types to be expressed quantitatively. The analysis of finger and palm prints is fully described in *The Genetics of Dermal Ridges* by Holt (1968). Essentially the method consists in counting the ridges on each finger according to defined rules, depending on the finger-print pattern, and then summing to give the total finger ridge-count. This quantity is almost entirely genetically determined, monozygotic twins differing in their total finger ridge-count no more than do the right and left hands of the same individual. However, the distributions of differences in total finger ridge-count in monozygotic and dizygotic twins overlap very considerably, so that half of the DZ twins have values in the range characteristic of MZ twins. The difference cannot therefore be used directly to make a zygosity diagnosis, but must be expressed as a probability. Several workers have derived discriminant functions of varying degrees of complexity to be used in this problem, and these are discussed critically by Holt (1968). They do not appear to offer substantial advantages over the simpler approach of Smith and Penrose who calculate the probability of dizygosity from the observed differences in total finger ridge-count in a series of twins of known zygosity. These values are listed in Table 2.11 and in any particular case the relative chance may be included in the calculation of zygosity along with the values for blood groups and other markers. The same approach can be used for another characteristic, the sum of the left and right maximal *atd* palmar angles (Table 2.12) again described fully by Holt (1968). Since this quantity is essentially independent of the total finger ridge-count, both these measures may be used in determining zygosity.

CONCLUSION

In summary, if twins are of unlike sex, then they are DZ. Similarly, pairs of twins with monochorionic placentation can be assumed to be MZ (Chapter 3) provided that the details of placental membrane relationships have been accurately recorded. However, if such data on placentation are not available, or in the case of dichorionic pairs of like sex, other studies will be necessary for the determination of zygosity. For this purpose it is preferable to use characters with a precise mode of inheritance such as red cell antigens, enzymes and other genetic markers in readily available tissues such as blood and placenta and then the probability of monozygosity or dizygosity can be calculated. In the case of a pair in which it is particularly important to be certain of zygosity, additional serological and biochemical tests can be performed in specialised laboratories. In adult twins similarity in physical appearance can also be used, but as the mode of inheritance of such characters is less well defined, this is a less satisfactory method as it is not possible to quantify the result exactly.

CHAPTER 3

Placentation

G. CORNEY

The placentation of twins shows a considerable degree of heterogeneity and can be responsible for profound effects on their intrauterine environment. It is therefore important, where possible, to take this situation into account when considering both an individual pair and also twin populations. Several monographs on twin placentation are available and particular features in these are: pathology (Benirschke and Driscoll, 1967), developmental aspects (Boyd and Hamilton, 1970) and early scientific work on the twin placenta (Gedda, 1961; Strong and Corney, 1967). The very comprehensive review on *Primary Biases in Twin Studies* by Price (1950) should perhaps be declared compulsory reading for the potential twin investigator, who should likewise take in the appreciation of twin studies by Allen (1965).

The form of the placentation of twins is probably most easily understood if viewed from the background of their origin. The *dizygotic* twinning process (Chapter 2) can be regarded as a duplication of the normal development of a single zygote; therefore, as might be expected, each member of a DZ pair has an individual placenta (Figure 2.1, page 18) with a chorionic and amniotic membrane, basically no different from that in a singleton pregnancy. This type of twin placentation is usually referred to as *dichorionic diamniotic*. The complications of morphology and of examination of such placentae after delivery arise only because various degrees of fusion of the placental discs sometimes take place, probably as a result of the proximity of implantation sites.

On the other hand, *monozygotic* twinning involves a highly abnormal sequence of events and it would not therefore seem strange if unusual forms of placentation were to be seen with this type of twinning; as will subsequently be described, this sometimes is the case. However, if division of the zygote takes place very early, close to the normal developmental schedule, a more conventional state of affairs exists and in terms of placentation the situation is essentially a duplication of the norm with two placentae (either separate or fused) and two chorionic and amniotic membranes. Atypical morphology appears, as might not unreasonably be expected, when unusual events take place, notably when the zygote has been 'programmed' to produce a single placenta which duly appears with its consequent chorionic membrane but with the programme in some disarray. The expected sequence, one placenta → one amniotic membrane→one embryo does not follow and duplication of the membranes (amniotic) and embryonic material takes place instead. These are however all variations on a single placental theme (Figure 2.3, page 21) and the placenta is always *monochorionic* (as with a normal singleton placenta) with internal variations such as two amnions (diamniotic) and two embryos or, more rarely, one amnion (monoamniotic) enclosing the two embryos in a single cavity.

It therefore follows that careful examination of the placentation of twins can produce valuable information about their origin.

EXAMINATION OF TWIN PLACENTAE

After delivery the placenta and membranes should be carefully examined as a considerable amount of information can be obtained from fairly simple procedures which might extend our knowledge about twinning in general and also about a particular pair (Benirschke, 1961). Twin placentation together with various recommendations for the technique of examination has been discussed fully together with the significance of normal and ab-normal findings by several authors in recent years (Benirschke and Driscoll, 1967; Strong and Corney, 1967; Cameron, 1968; Boyd and Hamilton, 1970) and for finer points of detail the interested reader would be advised to refer to these specialist publications. However, a general outline of the methodology will be given here.

UMBILICAL CORDS

The umbilical cords should be labelled at the time of delivery in some manner which will indicate which cord belonged to an individual twin. Elaborate procedures are often designed for this purpose, but in the case of twins it is really only necesssary to identify the cord of the first baby (special measures will of course be required in this respect for triplets or higher multiple births) and a convenient suggestion is that used by Edwards in the Birmingham Twin Study, namely that a safety pin (in a sterilised packet) is included on the delivery trolley and that this is inserted through the placental end of the cord of the first twin.

If samples of cord blood are required for studies of genetic markers or other investigations, they should be taken, preferably with a syringe and wide-bore needle to prevent contamination with maternal blood or Wharton's jelly, as soon as convenient after delivery. If there is to be delay in sending the blood for testing for genetic markers, the samples should be stored in a refrigerator (4 to 6°C) and not in a deep-freeze.

The position of insertion of the cords into the placenta should be recorded and also the number of vessels and any unusual features.

Velamentous insertion of the cord (that is when the cord originates from the chorion at some distance from the edge of the placenta), with consequent danger of rupture of fetal vessels, seems to be commoner in twins than in singletons and this applies particularly in the case of monochorionic twin placentation (Benirschke and Driscoll, 1967).

The absence of one umbilical artery appears to be commoner in twins than in singletons; Benirschke and Driscoll (1967) found this anomaly in 3.6 per cent of twins and the frequency in singletons is usually less than one per cent (Bryan and Kohler, 1974). As with singletons the presence of a single umbilical artery in a twin may be associated with congenital malformations in the baby, but there is a particular association with acardia (Benirschke, 1972a). It seems likely that there has been atrophy of one of the umbilical arteries and the cause might be linked with that of velamentous insertion of the cord. With the exception of acardia there does not seem to be a particular association with monozygotic twinning. The vessels in the cord usually spiral in an anti-clockwise manner (as in the case of singletons) but the direction of the spiral may differ between the twins (Edmonds, 1954).

TYPE OF PLACENTATION

The first and easiest observation to make is whether there are two placental masses or a single one. If there are two well defined, completely separate discs (Figure 3.1) then it follows, as has already been mentioned, that each will have a chorionic and an amniotic membrane and there will not, by definition, be any functional connection between them, i.e. no vascular communication. Thus the placentation is *dichorionic diamniotic* and the twin embryos, apart from sharing the same uterine environment, have been inde-pendent of each other.

However, if the placental mass is single or of indeterminate shape, more careful study is called for. The mass might be a single monochorionic placenta, or it might consist of two placentae (*dichorionic*) completely or partially fused (Figure 3.2 and 3.3). The differentiation between these various types can be found in the septum which divides the watery uterine environment of one embryo from that of his twin. Before examining the septum in detail, some guide to its expected membrane composition can be obtained from inspection of the fetal surface of the placenta. In the case of dichorionic placentae it seems likely that there is always a ridge running across this surface which is composed of two layers of chorion and is really the foundation of the chor-ionic 'wall' which separates the two cavities. It is not seen on the monochori-onic placenta which is usually completely smooth across the entire surface. This ridge is of very real help in differentiating the dichorionic from the mono-chorionic placenta and recognition of this feature should form part of the examination of all twin placentae (Bleisch, 1964; Nylander, 1970a). Too deep a significance (in vascular as well as metaphorical terms) should not be attached to the presence of this ridge, however. It does not necessarily denote the confines of the two underlying placental vascular territories (Figure 3.4) as radiological studies have shown (Strong and Corney, 1967) and injection studies are probably the only way in which the actual territories can be defined (Benirschke and Driscoll, 1967) though these are often not technically possible because the placenta has been torn at delivery.

The next step is to determine the number of membranes in the septum. The chorion tends to be more opaque than the amnion, but this appearance is not an infallible guide and most assistance in identification is gained by tracing the membranes down to the fetal surface of the placenta. The chorion, being an integral part of placental tissue, cannot be separated from it without

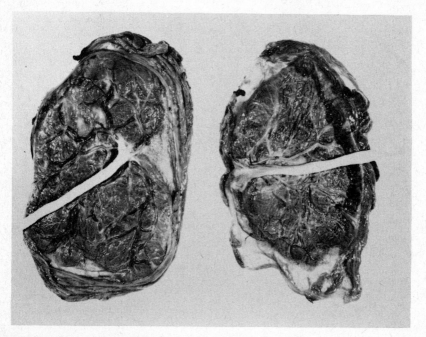

Figure 3.1. Separate dichorionic diamniotic placentae. From Strong and Corney (1967), with permission of Pergamon Press.

considerable difficulty; thus if the dividing septum of a completely or partially fused placenta is examined in this way, namely if the membranes are separated and traced down to the fetal surface, considerable resistance will be felt when the ridge mentioned previously is reached. Some degree of fusion of the chorionic membranes does occasionally take place (Bourne, 1962; Benirschke and Driscoll, 1967) which might make interpretation difficult, but if there is any doubt histological examination will confirm the true structure (Figure 3.5) of the septum. It has been speculated that chorionic fusion with subsequent disappearance of the dividing wall might occur in man; in other words a placenta, possibly associated with a DZ twin pair and originally destined to be dichorionic, would become monochorionic. This phenomenon is well known in other species (for discussion see Strong and Corney, 1967; Benirschke

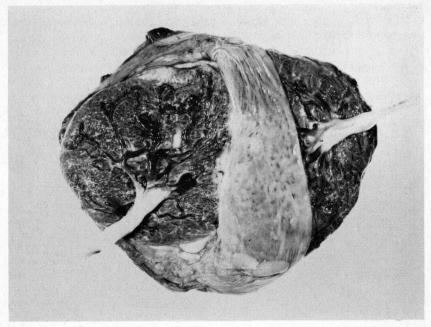

Figure 3.2. Fused dichorionic diamniotic placentae. From Strong and Corney (1967), with permission of Pergamon Press.

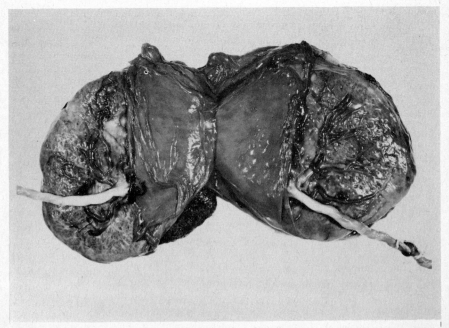

Figure 3.3. Partially fused dichorionic diamniotic placentae. From Strong and Corney (1967), with permission of Pergamon Press.

and Driscoll, 1967; Bulmer, 1970) but although some suspicious cases have been reported in man, many of them are not well substantiated. However, a well documented case has been reported recently by Nylander and Osunkoya (1970) in which unlike-sexed twins had what seemed to be at first inspection a monochorionic placenta, but on closer examination and at histology it was clear that there had originally been two complete layers of chorion in the dividing membrane but these had partially disappeared. Such a situation must

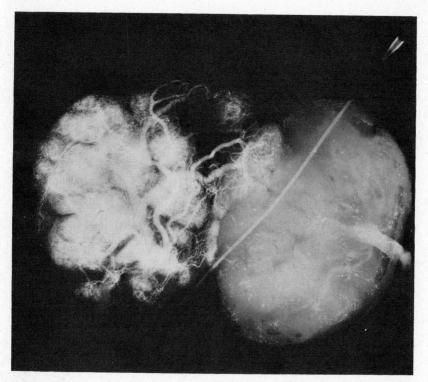

Figure 3.4. X-ray of fused dichorionic diamniotic placentae. One placenta has been injected with contrast medium and a catheter filled with the same material has been placed along the base of the septum. The junction of the vascular territories does not correspond to the insertion of the septum. From Strong and Corney (1967), with permission of Pergamon Press.

be extremely rare and is not likely to be a practical problem in routine obstetric practice.

In contrast to the chorion (Figures 3.6 and 3.7), the amnion is more transparent and also more friable. This membrane can easily be peeled away from the fetal aspect of the placenta (Benirschke, 1961; Bleisch, 1964) and this is the most critical test of differentiation from the chorion on macroscopic examination.

In summary, if the two adjacent membranes in the septum cannot be separated from the placenta, then two chorionic membranes are present. In such a case it automatically follows that there will also be two amniotic membranes, one for each chorion (*dichorionic diamniotic* placentation) and often quite closely adherent to its fetal surface, making separation difficult. A further possible source of confusion is the fact that the amnion might have been quite substantially torn away in the process of delivery. However, for precision an attempt should be made to identify all the four membranes which constitute the dividing 'wall' in fused dichorionic placentation. The often

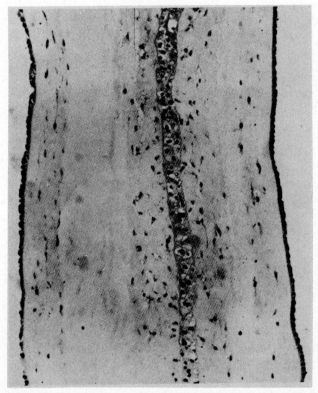

Figure 3.5. The dividing membrances of fused dichorionic diamniotic placentae. The two outer layers are composed of amnion. Between them the two layers of chorion have fused in the mid-line (H. & E., ×45). From Strong and Corney (1967), with permission of Pergamon Press.

somewhat arbitrary division of dichorionic diamniotic placentation into 'separate' and 'fused' categories is of doubtful biological significance as will be discussed later in this chapter and too much importance should not be attached to such morphological differences in this type of placentation.

If the main layers of the septum can be separated easily from the placental surface, then no chorionic tissue is present in the septum (which is composed of two amnia) and the only chorionic membrane is that surrounding the whole conceptus; the placentation in this case is *monochorionic diamniotic*.

There may, however, be no septum at all, the twins having shared the same amniotic cavity and there is only one amniotic membrane lining the enclosing chorionic sac. This, the rarest form of twin placentation, is *monochorionic monoamniotic*. This type of placentation might appear to be present if the amniotic membranes have been substantially torn away in the delivery process, but the clue to the true membrane structure can be found if a 'collar 'of

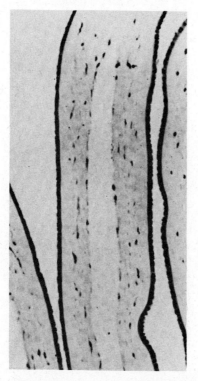

Figure 3.6. The dividing membranes of a monochorionic diamniotic placenta. Two layers of amnion with a potential space between them can be clearly seen (H. & E., ×45). From Strong and Corney (1967), with permission of Pergamon Press.

amnion remains at the base of the umbilical cords (Bleisch, 1964) indicating that two such membranes were originally present. A rare finding which might be of embryological significance is that of a fine line or 'plica' (Benirschke and Driscoll, 1967) extending across the surface of what seems to be a monoamniotic placenta. Sections of this area show two amnia whose tips are fused but do not show any epithelium suggesting previous scarring, possibly due to injury. Other similar reports are mentioned by these authors and they discuss possible reasons for this phenomenon. It seems likely that this might either be a remnant of a previous diamniotic septum which has at some stage during gestation been disrupted and subsequently almost disappeared, or that it represents a form of embryological-dating in that, if twinning had happened at the very moment when the amnion was forming, these membranes would be incomplete. Benirschke considers this latter hypothesis to be supporting evidence (Benirschke and Driscoll, 1967; Benirschke, 1972b) for his theory that the whole process of twinning should be regarded as a 'continuum'.

An examination along these lines is all that is required if the observer has experience in this field and the results can then be as accurate as histological examination (Nylander, 1970a). However, if such experience is lacking then either the findings should be confirmed by someone more knowledgeable, or specimens should be taken for histological examination. The most satisfactory

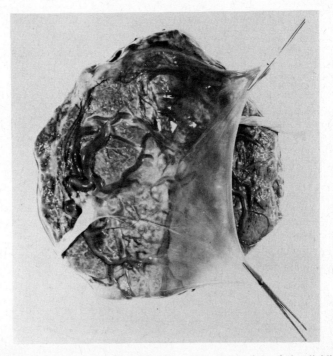

Figure 3.7. Monochorionic diamniotic placenta. The constitution of the dividing membranes, which are comparatively translucent, is amnion-amnion. From Strong and Corney (1967), with permission of Pergamon Press.

method of taking samples of the dividing membranes for histology is probably by taking a 'roll' of membranes with the aid of forceps; a segment (about 3 cm) can then be cut with scissors and placed in fixative (Benirschke and Driscoll, 1967; Benirschke, 1972b). This has been found to be more satisfactory by these authors than the alternative method, namely, taking a specimen including both membrane and placental tissue from the base of the septum ('T'-section method) which might, for example, prejudice future injection studies of placental vessels.

If the method of identifying the type of twin placentation has been accurate it is essential that the information should be recorded in the hospital notes, possibly accompanied by a diagram, in such a manner as to indicate that it has been reliably obtained. The data can then be used either for future studies of twin placentation or in determination of zygosity of a particular pair (in the case of monochorial placentation). This type of information would be extremely valuable as it has been found that retrospective information regarding twin placentation from hospital notes is usually open to considerable error, due to inaccurate interpretation of the findings (Benirschke, 1961; Benirschke and Driscoll, 1967; Nylander, 1970b). The weight of the placenta and any particular features should also be recorded. A photograph might be thought advisable if injection studies (discussed later in this chapter) have been performed or in the case of high multiple births. After examination, if injection studies are contemplated, they should be carried out as soon as convenient. If there is to be some delay, however, the placenta should be stored at 0 to 5°C. If enzyme studies on placental tissue for determination of zygosity are to be performed (see Chapter 2), a full-thickness block of placental tissue (about 10 g) should be taken from diametrically opposed sites. If quantitative studies (Aherne, Strong and Corney, 1968) of the component tissues of the placenta are planned, the weight and volume of the pieces of tissue removed should be recorded. After these various procedures have been completed the placenta should be placed in a suitable fixative (10 per cent formolsaline) if it is to be retained for further histological or other studies.

STUDIES OF TWIN PLACENTATION

As various forms of twin placentation are known to exist, it follows that many studies have been undertaken to determine the frequency of the different types in an attempt to obtain more information about the biological factors which might produce this deviation from the normal outcome of human pregnancy. Curiosity about the role of the placenta is probably as old as mankind and lack of detailed knowledge of this from earlier civilisations is presumably due to the absence of written information, though much has come to us from folklore and legend (Long, 1963). Certainly from the middle of the seventeenth century there is evidence (Strong and Corney, 1967) in European literature of a gathering interest in this aspect of twin births which gradually increased in momentum. This culminated in the middle decades of the nineteenth century with the monographs of Hueter (1845), Hyrtl (1870) and the monumental studies of Schatz over the last thirty years of that century which are summarised in his monograph published in 1900. These morphological studies form substantially more than the foundations of our knowledge of twin placentation today because although refinements have been added to their observations, further studies have in the main only confirmed both the findings of these workers and their opinions on the significance of them. Advances in knowledge about the biology of twinning in general, however, have been made possible by greater understanding (some of this because of newer techniques) of the physiology of pregnancy and also because of the subsequent emergence and application to reproductive biology, of genetical principles and methods of investigation. In the first fifty years of the present century this has consequently meant that twin studies could be carried out on a more formal basis and such investigations have included observations on newborn twins and their placentae. These investigations have been reviewed and discussed elsewhere (Strong and Corney, 1967; Benirschke and Driscoll, 1967; Boyd and Hamilton, 1970) and it is proposed now to discuss in detail only the findings from prospective studies which have been carried out in the last 10 to 15 years referring to the earlier workers only as seems appropriate. Similarly individual case reports will be quoted only if they illustrate some unusual aspect of a problem.

It is usually only possible to organise prospective studies of twin births in hospital as there are many problems associated with collection of samples from twin births at home. Fortunately a substantial number of twin deliveries take place in hospital and if a population sample is required, national or local population statistics might be available for comparison to determine if the sample is representative. However, it is not impossible to collect samples in addition from home deliveries, as was found in the Birmingham Twin Survey (Edwards, Cameron and Wingham, 1967—quoted in Strong and Corney, 1967, p. 38; Cameron, 1968) when specimens were obtained from well over 90 per cent of *all* twin births in the city. The key to success of this and other surveys carried out recently seems to be the availability of a very small number of personnel whose sole or main responsibility is the collection and subsequent examination of the samples of cord blood and placentae. Such persons do not necessarily need to have a high level of formal training as laboratory technicians because the basic techniques of placental membrane examination are quite simple as has already been explained. The results must however be reliable and it has been found highly satisfactory in the surveys carried out in Oxford (Corney, Robson and Strong, 1972) and in Nigeria (Nylander, 1970c) to use the services of a person without formal laboratory experience, but who had been trained in these particular techniques and whose sole responsibility this was. Naturally, more sophisticated studies such as histological examination or blood group studies must be carried out by specialist workers, but these results will be of little value if the samples have not been carefully collected, labelled and stored in the correct conditions.

The object of these recent surveys has been to study the relationship between the placentation and zygosity of twins, and those to be discussed took place in the United States (Benirschke, 1961; Potter, 1963; Fujikura and Froehlich, 1971), in England (Edwards, Cameron and Wingham, 1967; Cameron, 1968; Corney, Robson and Strong, 1972) and in Nigeria (Nylander, 1970c). Their organisation has been similar and in most cases a wide range of genetical markers has been tested, mainly in cord blood samples, but in some cases in placental tissue. Vascular injection studies have not been included in all of them and it has not been possible to continue such investigations in others as they are very time-consuming. The largest series to include injection studies is that from Birmingham (Cameron, 1968).

The results for the different types of placentation in these various surveys are given in Table 3.1. Apart from the higher proportion (30 per cent) of monochorionic pairs in the survey carried out by Benirschke (1961) and which is probably a reflection of the early gestational age (20 weeks) of some

Table 3.1. *Placentation of twin pairs in various populations.*

Country and reference	Ethnic group	Dichorionic	Monochorionic Diamniotic	Monochorionic Monoamniotic	Total
England					
Cameron (1968)[a]	Caucasian	534 (79.9%)	134 (20.1%)		668
Corney, Robson and Strong (1972)	Caucasian	405 (76.7%)	115 (21.8%)	8 (1.5%)	528
U.S.A.					
Benirschke (1961)	Caucasian	173 (69.2%)	74 (29.6%)	3 (1.2%)	250
Potter (1963)	Caucasian	431 (78.6%)	116 (21.2%)	1 (0.2%)	548
Fujikura and Froehlich (1971)	Caucasian	169 (75.6%)	52 (23.2%)	3 (1.3%)	224
	Negro	177 (76.6%)	47 (20.4%)	7 (3.0%)	231
Nigeria					
	Hausa (Northern Nigeria)	130 (87.8%)	18 (12.2%)	0	148
	Others (Northern Nigeria)	140 (87.5%)	20 (12.5%)	0	160
Nylander and Corney (1975)	Yoruba (Northern Nigeria)	146 (93.6%)	10 (6.4%)	0	156
Nylander (1970c)	Yoruba (Ibadan)	1361 (94.8%)	73 (5.1%)	2 (0.1%)	1436

[a] Figures estimated from percentage data in original publication.

of his cases, the findings amongst white populations in the United States and England are very similar. About 20 per cent of pairs have monochorionic placentation and this is of the same order as reported in earlier studies from Europe (for review see Strong and Corney, 1967) though some of these were rather small samples. The report by Cameron (1968) from the Birmingham Twin Survey does not include a separate classification for monochorionic monoamniotic placentation. However, in a subsequent publication (Wharton, Edwards and Cameron, 1968) 18 such cases (three per cent of all twins) were described. The single report from an American Negro population (Fujikura and Froehlich, 1971) shows a very similar proportion to that amongst Caucasians. The situation amongst the Yoruba people of Nigeria is however very different as only some five to six per cent of such pairs have a monochorionic placenta. The Hausa people and other ethnic groups in Northern Nigeria show a figure (12 per cent) intermediate between their Yoruba fellow-countrymen and European and North American populations. At present there are no other data of this type available from Africa or from any other part of the world and other comparisons cannot therefore be made. Such information would be of great interest however and the search for it need not necessarily involve very complex techniques. As has been stated previously, the examination of the placenta is quite simple from the point of view of determining the membrane relationships. The ability to recognise a monochorionic placenta can be learnt after very little tuition and, as has been discussed, observation of the 'ridge' appears to be reliable in identifying dichorionic placentae. Injection studies are unnecessary for the confirmation of monochorial status and if the observer is reliable it seems that histological studies are not required. Thus where these facilities are not available (Nylander, 1970a) simple macroscopic examination is probably adequate and well suited to population studies. Moreover, as will be discussed later in this chapter, since all studies so far reported have shown that all twins with a monochorionic placenta are alike in sex and all genetic markers tested (and are probably therefore monozygotic) it would now seem reasonable to say that if such a placenta has been examined by a reliable observer, it is no longer essential to test for a wide range of genetic markers in cord blood. This would certainly not seem to be necessary for population studies. Nylander (1970d) has also shown from data published for the United Kingdom and the U.S.A. that there is an inverse relationship between the twinning rate and the proportion of monochorionic pairs in a population. In other words if the twinning rate is high, as amongst the Yoruba in Nigeria, then the proportion of monochorionic twins is low. This is because the racial differences in twinning rates seem to be due to differences in the proportions of DZ twins (Bulmer, 1970), the MZ twinning rate remaining constant. Nylander (1970d) has suggested that it would be interesting to observe if this relationship between the proportion of monochorionic placentae and the twinning rate in a population also applies in other parts of the world.

PLACENTATION AND ZYGOSITY

As has already been discussed in Chapter 2, it was originally theoretically supposed over fifty years ago that some MZ twins might have individual (dichorionic) as opposed to shared (monochorionic) placentation. This was not, however, confirmed until studies of twins of known placentation were made during the 1930s comparing various physical characteristics and also using the then relatively novel technique of blood group determination (for discussion see Price, 1950). Since then the emergence or, one might say, explosion, of numerous other genetic markers has led to greater precision in the determination of zygosity, as has also been explained in the previous chapter, and it has therefore been possible to examine the placentae of new-born twins of known zygosity for their membrane relationships. The efficiency of zygosity determination by these techniques will depend upon both the number of markers used and also their value (in other words the amount of genetic variation which they display) in a particular population which is being studied. For example, AK (adenylate kinase) is a useful enzyme marker in English populations but is not helpful in Nigeria and in the case of Pep A (peptidase A) the reverse applies.

Some idea of the efficiency of such a system for determination of zygosity in population studies can be gained from examination of the results from pairs of unlike sex who are therefore known to be DZ and would be expected to show some differences between the genetic markers studied. An illustration of this is provided by the Nigerian sample in Table 3.2 in which such

Table 3.2. *Results of typing 455 pairs of Nigerian twins for a set of genetic markers.*

		Total pairs	Markers same	Markers different
Dichorionic	Same sex	250	54	196
	Different sex	188	30	158
Monochorionic	Same sex	17	17	0
	Different sex	0	0	0
		455	101	354

From Nylander and Corney (1969), with permission of the editors of *Annals of Human Genetics* and Cambridge University Press.

differences were found amongst only 196 of the 250 pairs of unlike sex. The system used was not therefore very efficient for detecting DZ pairs. However, on the assumption that a similar degree of inefficiency would also operate amongst pairs of *like* sex, Edwards (Edwards, Cameron and Wingham, 1967) suggested a formula which, by taking account of the numbers of pairs differing in markers amongst those of known zygosity (i.e., unlike sex) would allow an estimation to be made of the true number of DZ pairs of like sex. This formula was subsequently modified by Nylander (Nylander and Corney, 1969) and a note on the estimation of the standard errors by C. A. B. Smith

is provided in the same publication. The method is perhaps best illustrated
by an example with reference to Table 3.2.

The sample of twins in Table 3.2 is divided up as follows:

Total number of pairs $t = 455$

Dichorionic $d = 438$

Monochorionic (same sex assumed to be monozygotic) $m = 17$	Same sex $s = 250$		Unlike sex $u = 188$	
	Alike in all markers $A = 54$	Different in some markers $B = 196$	Alike in all markers $a = 30$	Different in some markers $b = 158$

Among $u = 188$ pairs known to be dizygotic, there are $b = 158$ which differ
in at least one marker. Hence, by using the same proportion, since there are
$B = 196$ pairs of the same sex which differ in at least one marker, one can
estimate that there are altogether

$$r = Bu/b = 233.2$$

dizygotic pairs of the same sex. There are s dichorionic pairs of the same sex,
and taking away r dizygotic, there remains $(s-r)$ monozygotic. Hence among
all d dichorionic pairs, a proportion

$$z = (s - r)/d = 0.038$$

are estimated to be monozygotic. And among all the monozygotic pairs,
which are estimated to number $(m + s - r) = 33.7$, a proportion

$$y = (s - r)/(m + s - r) = 0.50$$

are estimated to be dichorionic.

Thus the actual number of DZ pairs of like sex is 233 (196 in the original
testing). Similarly the number of MZ (dichorionic) pairs is 17 (in contrast to
54 pairs who were alike for markers tested). In other words 37 pairs of twins
were originally classified as alike when they were in fact DZ. The system
originally used for determination of zygosity was therefore not very efficient.

The results of recent newborn twin population studies in England, the
United States and Nigeria are shown in Tables 3.3 and 3.4, correction for
inefficiency of the markers having been applied (according to the method just
described) as noted at the foot of the tables.

As has been known for many years, the majority of twins are DZ and a
minority MZ. From the distribution of like and unlike-sexed pairs and using
the Weinberg formula (see Chapter 5) it has been previously established
(for review see Bulmer, 1970) that the variation in the twinning rate throughout the world is due to the numbers of DZ twins and the findings in the newborn populations studied by genetic markers and shown in Table 3.3 are, in
general, consistent with those estimated by the Weinberg method. Thus about
70 per cent of twins in England and the U.S.A. are DZ, whereas more than
90 per cent are derived from two zygotes amongst the Yorubas in Nigeria.
The somewhat anomalous finding of a smaller proportion of DZ twins amongst

Table 3.3. *Zygosity of twin pairs in various populations.*

| | England | | U.S.A. | | | Nigeria | | | |
| | Edwards, Cameron & Wingham (1967)[a] | Corney, Robson & Strong (1972)[b] | Potter (1963)[a] | Fujikura & Froehlich (1971)[b] | | | Nylander & Corney (1975)[c] | | Nylander (1970c)[c] |
	Caucasian	Caucasian	Caucasian	Caucasian	Negro	Hausa	Others	Yoruba (N. Nigeria)	Yoruba (Ibadan)
MZ	163 (27.5%)	151 (28.6%)	105 (35.8%)	71 (36.4%)	80 (39.2%)	11 (17.7%)	20 (26.3%)	3 (4.5%)	120 (8.4%)
DZ	429 (72.5%)	377 (71.4%)	188 (64.2%)	124 (63.6%)	124 (60.8%)	51 (82.3%)	56 (73.7%)	63 (95.5%)	1316 (91.6%)
Total	592	528	293	195	204	62	76	66	1436

[a] Corrected for inefficiency of markers from original data according to method explained in text.
[b] Markers sufficiently efficient to require no further correction.
[c] Corrected for inefficiency of markers in the original papers.

Table 3.4. *Placentation and zygosity of twin pairs in various populations.*

Country	Reference	Ethnic group	Dichorionic		Monochorionic		Total
			MZ	DZ	MZ	DZ	
England	Edwards, Cameron and Wingham (1967)[a]	Caucasian	47	429	116	0	592
	Corney, Robson and Strong (1972)[b]	Caucasian	28	377	123	0	528
U.S.A.	Potter (1963)[a]	Caucasian	38	188	67	0	293
	Fujikura and Froehlich (1971)[b]	Caucasian	16	124	55	0	195
		Negro	26	124	54	0	204
Nigeria		Hausa	4	51	7	0	62
		Others	8	56	12	0	76
	Nylander and Corney (1975)[c]	Yoruba (Northern Nigeria)	0	63	3	0	66
	Nylander (1970c)[c]	Yoruba (Ibadan)	45	1316	75	0	1436

[a],[b],[c] See footnotes to Table 3.3.

Table 3.5. *Dichorionic placentation and zygosity in various populations.*

Country	Reference	Ethnic group	Total no. of pairs	Percentage of MZ twins who are dichorionic	Percentage of dichorionic twins who are MZ
England	Edwards, Cameron and Wingham (1967)[a]	Caucasian	592	28.8	9.9
	Corney, Robson and Strong (1972)[b]	Caucasian	528	18.5	6.9
U.S.A.	Potter (1963)[a]	Caucasian	293	36.2	16.8
	Fujikura and Froehlich (1971)[b]	Caucasian	195	22.5	11.4
		Negro	204	32.5	17.3
Nigeria	Nylander (1970c)[c]	Yoruba	1436	37.5	3.3

[a], [b], [c] See footnotes to Table 3.3.

Negroes than amongst Caucasians in the survey from North America described by Fujikura and Froehlich (1971) could be due to the small size of the populations studied. Population data from the U.S.A. (Shipley et al, 1967; Heuser, 1967) show the reverse trend, namely that, as expected, there is a slightly higher proportion of DZ twins amongst Negroes (than amongst Caucasians).

Twins with monochorionic placentation in each survey (Table 3.4) have consistently been alike in sex and all markers tested and it therefore now seems reasonable to say with confidence that (if examined by a reliable observer) this form of placentation can be taken to indicate monozygosity. In the case of dichorionic placentation the majority of twins are DZ, but a minority, as had previously been supposed and to some extent verified, are probably MZ. It is not surprising that no dichorionic MZ pairs were found amongst the Yorubas in Northern Nigeria (Nylander and Corney, 1975); the sample is only a small one and as the MZ twinning rate in that population is very low (Nylander, 1971b), very few, if any, MZ dichorionic pairs would have been expected in a sample of this size. Further details with regard to dichorionic placentation and zygosity are given in Table 3.5. The proportion of MZ twins with dichorionic placentation varies quite widely between the different surveys, but it would seem to lie between 20 and 40 per cent. Alternatively, in a sample of dichorionic pairs there would be expected to be very few (three per cent) MZ Yoruba twins in Nigeria as compared with Caucasians (10 to 17 per cent) in England or the U.S.A.

DICHORIONIC PLACENTAL FORM AND ZYGOSITY

Dichorionic placentae can either be *separate* or *fused* and this additional classification is given in some, but not all, of the reports from prospective surveys. However, the criteria are not always very clearly defined; for example, in the Oxford study (Corney, Robson and Strong, 1972) such placentae were said to be fused when the two placental discs were adherent to each other and separate when they could be parted quite easily, whereas Fujikura and Froehlich (1971) included in the 'separate' category those in which the membranes were 'loosely adherent'. Potter (1963) defined fused placentae as those which could not be individually delineated by simple inspection and 'double' (termed separate by others) placentation as the situation when the two were separate, easily distinguishable masses. Such criteria are obviously open to differences in interpretation and whilst the findings might be consistent within a particular survey, it makes comparison of results between surveys difficult, for example, with regard to the possible effect on birth weight (Corney, Robson and Strong, 1972). For the same reasons it would be unwise to pool such data. It has been claimed by Fujikura and Froehlich (1971) that monozygosity is more frequent amongst twins with fused placentae than amongst those with individual placentation. The reason for this is thought to be that after early division of a single zygote, the two masses of cells would inevitably pass down the same Fallopian tube and would therefore

Table 3.6. *Form of dichorionic placentation of twin pairs in various populations.*

Country and reference	Ethnic group	Dichorionic		Monochorionic	Total
		Fused	Separate		
England					
Strong and Corney (1967)	Caucasian	66 (33.7%)	85 (43.4%)	45 (22.9%)	196
Corney, Robson and Strong (1972)	Caucasian	141 (26.9%)	261 (49.7%)	123 (23.4%)	525[a]
U.S.A.					
Benirschke (1961)	Caucasian	85 (34.0%)	88 (35.2%)	77 (30.8%)	250
Potter (1963)	Caucasian	192 (35.0%)	239 (43.6%)	117 (21.4%)	548
Fujikura and Froehlich (1971)	Caucasian	100 (44.6%)	69 (30.8%)	55 (24.6%)	224
	Negro	106 (45.9%)	71 (30.7%)	54 (23.4%)	231
Nigeria					
Nylander (1970c)	Yoruba	754 (52.5%)	607 (42.3%)	75 (5.2%)	1436

[a] The form of dichorionic placentation was not known in three pairs (Table 3.1).

be more likely to implant in close proximity on the wall of the uterus. This is a reasonable hypothesis, but as the whole argument revolves around the question of 'fusion' or 'separation' the criteria are very important.

The data from those surveys in which this type of information is provided are shown in Table 3.6. That from the Oxford survey is given in two forms (Strong and Corney, 1967; Corney, Robson and Strong, 1972) as some of the early cases in the 1967 series have not been included in the final analysis of this survey in 1972 because fewer genetic markers were available at the beginning of the survey. Moreover, whilst there was only a single observer for the type of placentation in the 1967 series, there were two additional observers for the rest of the survey. The form of placentation was recorded by a single person in the Nigerian series (Nylander, 1970c) and it would seem likely that such observations were probably uniform in the surveys described by Benirschke and Potter, but the data reported by Fujikura and Froehlich were obtained from a number of different hospitals and it is presumably therefore possible that there might have been some variation in interpretation of the criteria for the form of dichorionic placentation. Amongst the various results shown in Table 3.6 there are approximately equal proportions of fused and separate dichorionic placentae, but there is a not inconsiderable degree of variation between the surveys which presumably reflects different interpretations of the criteria and this makes it difficult to draw other conclusions, for example, with regard to the possible effect of zygosity on placental form.

However, in order to examine the hypothesis that cell masses from a single zygote might give rise more often to fused dichorionic placentae, the requisite information from the various surveys is given in Table 3.7. Two of the surveys in Table 3.6 have been excluded, notably those of Benirschke (1961) for which information on zygosity determined by genetic markers is not available and of Strong and Corney (1967) where the system used for determination of zygosity was not considered efficient enough to be informative in this type of analysis. It can be seen that, apart from the results of Corney, Robson and Strong (1972), there is in general a higher proportion of fused placentae amongst MZ pairs than amongst DZ pairs, which would favour the hypothesis. However, in view of the variation in criteria for dichorionic placental form, this observation should probably be viewed with some caution.

There seems therefore to be little justification for attempting to include observations on such variations in dichorionic placental form as part of the routine examination of the placenta in the delivery room. Precision in such circumstances can hardly be achieved if the results in carefully mounted surveys are as variable as seems to be the case. It is suggested therefore that emphasis should be placed on differentiation between dichorionic and monochorionic placentae. It has often been the custom to use the terms 'uniovular' (monochorionic) and 'binovular' (dichorionic) when describing twin placentation particularly in hospital notes. Whether the former (uniovular) continues to be used is a matter of personal preference, but 'binovular' is inaccurate and should be discarded. Both terms imply that the zygosity is known from placental examination and it would be more accurate to substitute the descriptive terms 'monochorionic' and 'dichorionic' when recording the type of twin placentation.

Table 3.7. *Form of dichorionic placentation and zygosity of twin pairs in various populations.*

Country and reference	Ethnic group	MZ dichorionic				DZ dichorionic				Zygosity not known	Total
		Fused	Separate	Total	%Fused	Fused	Separate	Total	%Fused		
England Corney, Robson and Strong (1972)[b]	Caucasian	8	20	28	28.6	133	241	374	35.6	0	402
U.S.A. Potter (1963)[a]	Caucasian	20	18	38	52.6	81	107	188	43.1	0	226
Fujikura and Froehlich (1971)[b]	Caucasian	14	2	16	87.5	66	58	124	53.2	29	169
	Negro	22	4	26	84.6	68	56	124	54.8	27	177
Nigeria Nylander (1970c)[c]	Yoruba	40	5	45	88.9	714	602	1316	54.3	0	1361

[a], [b], [c] See footnotes to Table 3.3.

In summary, whilst a monochorionic placenta is of considerable help in determination of zygosity, no assistance can be gained in this respect from dichorionic placentation and in the case of like-sexed twins with this form of placentation, further studies by genetic markers will be needed to determine zygosity. For example, in England some 33 per cent of twins are of unlike sex, and are therefore DZ; a further 20 per cent (all of which will be of like sex) have monochorionic placentation and are almost certain to be MZ. Thus in a sample of English twins, whilst the zygosity of some 53 per cent can be determined by sex or examination of the placental membranes, other studies will be required for the remaining (47 per cent) dichorionic pairs of like sex.

VASCULAR COMMUNICATIONS

A further differentiation between dichorionic and monochorionic twin placentation, and one which can have far-reaching implications in both structural and functional terms for the twin babies, is the fact that monochorionic pairs have a common placental circulation whilst dichorionic pairs are independent of each other in this respect. There are exceptions to both situations, but they are probably rare and it can usually be assumed that the majority of MZ pairs have had a common (though not, as will be discussed, necessarily similar) placental blood supply in utero whereas DZ twins and a minority of MZ pairs (i.e., those with dichorionic placentation) have not. In other words, the intrauterine environment of DZ and MZ dichorionic pairs is in this respect similar, but differs from that of (MZ) monochorionic pairs. In the former category individual twins might have differing environmental influences such as sites of implantation and discordant responses to intra-uterine infections, but in the latter group intra-pair differences, for example, in birth weight and some malformations, are more likely to be due to a unique cause, namely inequalities in the common placental circulation (Price, 1950; Gruenwald, 1970).

The anatomical aspects of such vascular communications have been studied in depth in the last hundred years or so, and details can be found in several monographs (Hyrtl, 1870; Schatz, 1900a; Benirschke and Driscoll, 1967; Strong and Corney, 1967; Boyd and Hamilton, 1970). How they are formed is still a mystery. Observations of morphology have often been carefully recorded, but not infrequently these have been accompanied by a tremendous amount of speculation about the mechanism of subsequent derangements of blood flow and it must be remembered that we are still largely ignorant about the physiological (or to be precise pathophysiological) facts of the situation. One possibly informative line of research which surprisingly seems not to have been followed is systematic perfusion under physiological conditions of the freshly delivered monochorionic twin placenta, and until experiments on this or other similar lines (possibly in animals) are performed, it is difficult to see how we can better understand the mechanism of intrauterine competition for placental blood supply in some twin pregnancies.

IDENTIFICATION OF VASCULAR COMMUNICATIONS

There are two main types of such anastomoses, those which are superficial, in other words on the fetal surface of the placenta and those which are deep in the substance of the organ. The former which can easily be identified by naked eye (Figure 3.8) are between arteries or between veins, whereas the latter connect artery and vein and take place by way of a cotyledon. These arteriovenous communications which Schatz (see Price, 1950, for discussion) termed 'areas of villous transfusion' (Figure 3.9) constitute what he termed

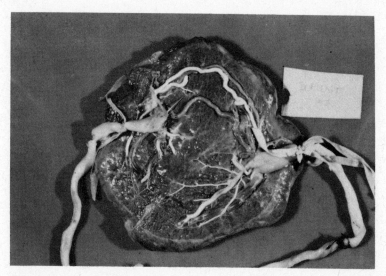

Figure 3.8. Monochorionic diamniotic placenta. The vessels of twin 2 (right) have been injected and the vessels of the other twin have filled through both arterial and venous anastomoses. From Strong and Corney (1967), with permission of Pergamon Press.

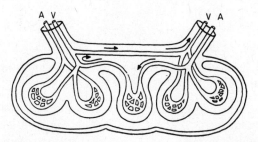

Figure 3.9. A schematic representation of the vascular anastomoses in the normal monochorionic twin placenta, based on the ideas of Schatz. An arteriovenous anastomosis is depicted in the centre of the placenta, fed by an artery from the right and drained by a vein to the left. The blood is restored to its proper route by the superficial vein-vein anastomosis. From Aherne et al (1968) *Biologia Neonatorum*, **13**, 121, by permission of S. Karger AG, Basel.

the *third circulation* (the other two being the circulatory system of each twin). They are frequently multiple and are to be found along the equator separating the individual territories of a monochorionic twin placenta (Figure 3.10). In each area the artery (Figure 3.10) can be seen to disappear into the placenta, the equivalent vein emerging a short distance away; the areas are often quite small, but assistance in identification can be gained from the fact that the

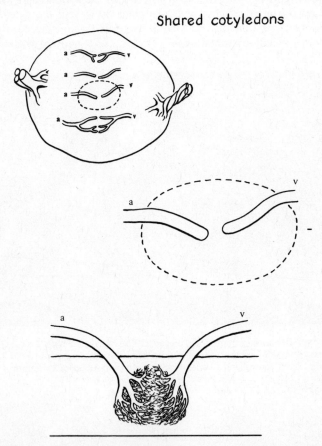

Shared cotyledons

Figure 3.10. Diagram illustrating the general appearance and distribution of arteriovenous communications in a monochorionic twin placenta.

artery leading to the cotyledon is not, as is customary, accompanied by a vein. Similarly the emergent vein is not paired with an artery on its course across the placental surface.

However, whilst some attempt might be made to identify such communications by naked eye, this is not entirely reliable in either qualitative or quantitative terms, for example, arteries usually cross superficial to veins, but this is not invariable (Bhargava, Chakravarty and Raja, 1971) and cannot be relied upon for identification of the type of vessel (i.e., artery or vein). Most workers agree that some form of injection study is a better method and it is generally thought that the presence of vascular communications cannot otherwise be excluded. Over the years numerous media including air, milk, red wine (shame !) and many other materials of diverse colour and consistency have been used. In recent years refinements have been introduced including radio-opaque materials with subsequent x-ray studies (Strong and Corney, 1967; Aherne, Strong and Corney, 1968) and also various corrosion techniques (Bhargava, Chakravarty and Raja, 1971), the latter yielding very beautiful specimens, but possibly not being very informative in terms of functional communication. If the intention is to demonstrate that fluid (and by implication therefore, blood) can pass from one side of the placenta to the other, and if so at what points and by what type of vessels, then possibly the

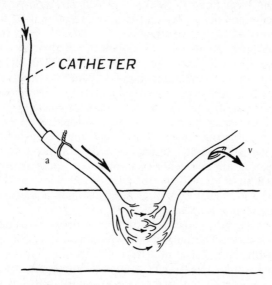

Figure 3.11. Diagram illustrating the technique for the injection of shared cotyledons (arteriovenous communications).

simplest and most informative method is to inject coloured saline (Benirschke, 1961). This is a simple technique which can easily be carried out with a syringe in the delivery room; the whole placenta can be washed out by means of a catheter inserted into the vessels of the umbilical cord. If there is delay in carrying out the examination, or if the placenta has been torn at delivery, selected areas of the placenta can be used for catheterisation (Figure 3.11) and the subsequent course of the injected fluid observed with the naked eye. Such a 'look and see what happens' approach is probably better than more complex methods which need a lot more preparation and interpretation and are far removed from the physiological situation anyway. A discussion of various methods is given by Benirschke and Driscoll (1967) and Strong and Corney (1967). Whilst experience in identifying superficial communications can be gained quite quickly, the arteriovenous areas require more practice as some of them can be quite small, are easily overlooked and are also more difficult to catheterise.

It is obviously impractical to include such investigations in the routine examination of the placenta but if such study is made, it is useful to have a photograph of the placenta or possibly a sketch or diagram. There is in any case something to be said for routinely making a sketch of twin placentae in the hospital notes.

VASCULAR COMMUNICATIONS IN MONOCHORIONIC DIAMNIOTIC PLACENTAE

The largest series in which injection techniques have been used is that from the Birmingham Twin Survey, details of which are reported by Cameron (1968) and experience there was that it was exceptional to find a monochorionic placenta without anastomoses. This has also been the experience of other workers (for discussion and review see Benirschke and Driscoll, 1967; Strong and Corney, 1967; Boyd and Hamilton, 1970) all of whom have found that some form of communication was usually present with this type of placentation. In a few cases, however, none could be demonstrated and this failure does not seem simply to be due to lack of experience as considerable expertise had often been acquired by the time such placentae were examined. It is of course possible that anastomoses might have been present earlier in gestation but had subsequently disappeared. It can therefore be said that, except very rarely, all monochorionic placentae possess some form of anastomosis and since, as will be discussed, dichorionic placentae do not, then the observation of such communicating channels is useful confirmatory evidence of monochorionic placentation.

They do, however, vary enormously in type, number, size and presumably therefore, in function. The commonest combination seems to be that of artery–artery with some form of arteriovenous (i.e., artery–vein and/or vein–artery) connection. Vein–vein communications are rare. When the superficial anastomoses (artery–artery or vein–vein) are either very small or absent it is thought that an imbalance occurs in the common circulation of the twins with deleterious effects. This hypothesis that the superficial anastomoses act as a compensatory mechanism for the deep arteriovenous communications was originally put forward by Friedrich Schatz, a German obstetrician, in a series of papers between 1875 and the end of the nineteenth century (for review see Price, 1950; Benirschke and Driscoll, 1967; Strong and Corney, 1967) and summarised in his monograph in 1900. It must, however, be remembered, as he emphasised, that numerous other variables such as torsion of the cord, primary defects of the fetal heart and problems at delivery might also operate and it is likely that the resultant effect on the twins (the so-called 'twin-transfusion syndrome') is not solely due to the presence of anastomoses. Many of these other factors cannot be demonstrated after delivery but they might, in major part, account for malfunction within the common circulation leading to the death of many twins. Amazingly little has been added in the last hundred years to our knowledge of this particular and not inconsiderable area of fetal morbidity and mortality. There is no lack of morphological information but on the functional aspect we are still more or less in the nineteenth century.

THE PLACENTA IN THE TWIN-TRANSFUSION SYNDROME

The appearance of the placenta can be quite helpful in making the diagnosis particularly if the babies are stillborn and other investigations are not therefore possible. In some cases there may be a very marked difference in the colour of the maternal surface (Herlitz, 1941; Benirschke and Driscoll, 1967; Aherne, Strong and Corney, 1968), that of the 'donor' being large and pale, not dissimilar to that in Rhesus blood group incompatibility, and that of the 'recipient' small and congested. Histological studies show that chorionic villi in the donor territory are bulky and oedematous with thicker trophoblast than is found in the case of the recipient. Chorionic villi in the recipient twin's territory are normal in size and configuration, but the fetal vessels are dilated and congested. Fetal capillaries in the donor portion are small in calibre and often contain nucleated red cell precursors. Morphometric studies by Aherne (Aherne, Strong and Corney, 1968) have shown that the chorionic villous surface area is about twice as great in the donor as in the recipient territory but there is no villous hyperplasia and it is thought that these appearances are solely due to the oedema, though the reason for this is unknown. Fetal capillaries in the donor territory are only half as wide but are several times longer than those of the recipient and this in conjunction with other factors would tend to slow blood flow in this territory with, possibly, a consequent adverse effect on fetal nutrition. Aherne also found that within the cotyledon in affected cases there is variation in the size of the vessels, some having normal structure, others being reduced in calibre and such changes might, according to the direction of flow, presumably play a very important part in determining the outcome for the twin babies.

Extensive morphological changes of this type in both fetus and placenta would imply that the process has been going on for some time during the pregnancy. The timing of the 'transfusion' from one twin into the other has been the subject of debate in many papers but presumably, as with many other aspects of this strange phenomenon, there is no single answer. Many authors have felt that the whole episode takes place at delivery and it has been suggested (Klebe and Ingomar, 1972) that in cases where there is only a small difference in birth weight, in other words intrauterine nutrition has probably not been affected, then the delivery process might be the 'trigger' which initiates the cross-transfusion. However, in other cases there is much evidence apart from body-weight difference, in favour of a natural history possibly extending throughout the whole of pregnancy. Hydramnios can occur during pregnancy in association with this syndrome (Benirschke and Driscoll, 1967) the excess fluid usually being in the amniotic sac of the recipient twin. Nucleated red cells may also be seen in the blood of the donor (Herlitz, 1941; Strong and Corney, 1967) the clinical picture in this twin often bearing a close resemblance to 'erythroblastosis fetalis' due to blood group incompatibility. A discrepancy in heart size has been observed between twins whose approximate gestational age was only 10 weeks (Benirschke, 1972a; Benirschke and Kim, 1973) and it was presumed that this was not the result of a recent event. Naeye (1965) has reported very detailed studies on the organs of affected twins and has shown, as did Schatz, that there are very marked quantitative differences, for example cardiac hypertrophy in the recipient twin, and he has suggested that hypertension might be present, but studies to confirm or refute this have not been reported. The kidneys may also show interesting changes particularly in the recipient, as the glomeruli can be very much enlarged and also appear more mature. It is thought that increased glomerular filtration in association with increased blood volume and pressure accounts certainly in part for the excess amniotic fluid in the sac of this baby (Naeye, 1963). The exact mechanism for the production of hydramnios in this setting is not however fully understood (Benirschke and Driscoll, 1967) and may in some measure be due to materno-fetal transfer of fluid (Klooster-man, 1963). The organs of the donor twin are usually below the expected size and this presumably reflects a severe degree of malnutrition (Naeye, 1965). How this happens is not clear; Kloosterman (1963) has pointed out that the communicating channels are sometimes very small and it is therefore difficult to understand how appreciable amounts of blood could be transferred. He suggests that the more important factor in the causation of discrepant growth in the donor and hydramnios in the sac of the recipient is likely to be the demonstrable intra-pair differences in plasma proteins. Hyperproteinaemia in the recipient might, for example, as a result of differences in osmotic pressures, encourage transfer of fluid from the mother to the fetus. Plasma protein values have occasionally been included in individual case reports, but the matter has not been specifically studied until recently. In a case of the transfusion syndrome, Bryan and Slavin (1974) found that the level of cord serum immunoglobin G (IgG) in the donor twin was very much lower than in the recipient. This discrepancy was far greater than in the case of the total protein, albumin, transferrin and alpha-1-antitrypsin. A similar discrepancy of IgG values was found in two further pairs and subsequently in three additional cases of the transfusion syndrome (Bryan, 1975). As IgG in the newborn is the only protein of maternal origin it is suggested that there might be some disturbance of materno-fetal transfer of IgG in the case of the donor twin (Bryan and Slavin, 1974) This is of interest in view of the earlier indication (Aherne, Strong and Corney, 1968) that, in addition to possible transport delays within the placenta, the structural changes in the chorion of the donor twin might reduce the efficiency with which substances are transferred from maternal to fetal blood.

It is also possible, as was in general postulated by Herlitz (1941) and subsequently more specifically by Walker and Turnbull (1955) and Naeye (1963) that some substance such as erythropoietin produced as a response to anaemia in the donor might incidentally also stimulate the other twin.

Thus most, if not all, monochorionic twins have some form of common circulation which will in some way play havoc with intrauterine existence for many of them and some will not survive, but why this should happen is ill-understood. It certainly seems that in many cases it is not just a simple shift of blood from one to the other as has so often been implied. There is room for a great deal of further investigation possibly along different lines than the traditional 'shunting' approach and there might then be some hope of reaching a destination.

Monoamniotic placentae

The discussion with regard to vascular communications has been mainly with regard to monochorionic diamniotic placentae. The situation is less clear with regard to monochorionic monoamniotic placentae; it would seem likely that the same situation would apply, namely that most, if not all, would have some form of anastomosis, but this is not certain. As such placentae only form some one to three per cent of all twin placentae (Table 3.1) naturally there are few reports of injection studies; however, Hyrtl (1870) thought that anastomoses were present 'without exception' in such placentae. More recently Wharton, Edwards and Cameron (1968) from cases seen in the Birmingham Twin Survey, found such communications in 16 out of 18 placentae studied and presumed (as one of the twins was acardiac, see below) that they would have been found in another had full studies been possible. Bhargava, Chakravarty and Raja (1971) demonstrated anastomoses in all six monoamniotic placentae studied. However, Benirschke and Driscoll (1967) describe a case in which no definite anastomoses were seen and quote Wenner (1956) as saying that 'Siamese twins' (who would be expected to have this type of placentation) might not always have anastomoses. However, Boyd and Hamilton (1970) found such communications in the two monoamniotic placentae each from conjoined twins (thoracopagus) which they studied. Strong and Corney (1967) did not find any anastomoses in the single monoamniotic placenta which they examined. Thus it seems, as with the monochorionic diamniotic type that vascular communications may not always be present; there are not enough reports available to indicate precisely how often this happens, but on present data it would seem to be in a minority of cases. Additional evidence in favour of the presence of communicating channels can be found in the occasional reports of the transfusion syndrome in monoamniotic twins (Meyer, Keith and Webster, 1970; Hollander, 1969) and also in the gross anomaly known as *acardia*.

Acardia

As the name implies, in this fetal malformation there is no heart; it is found only in multiple pregnancies and, in humans, in those arising from a single zygote. The frequency is of the order of one in 100 MZ twins (Napolitani and Schreiber, 1960). However, acardia is thought to form part of a group of malformations which includes many other aberrations of development such as absence of the head (acephaly) and formless masses which, whilst containing fetal parts, cannot be identified as a baby. Many exercises in classification of these malformations have been carried out, but these are probably somewhat meaningless as their pathogenesis is probably similar (Benirschke and Kim, 1973).

VASCULAR COMMUNICATIONS IN DICHORIONIC PLACENTAE

The situation here is quite different as anastomoses are certainly unusual and probably very rare. In the older literature reports appeared from time to time, but some are of rather dubious value (for review and discussion see Price, 1950; Benirschke and Driscoll, 1967; Strong and Corney, 1967) for example because of the technique used or ambiguous interpretation of the findings. However, anastomoses have been clearly demonstrated twice by Cameron in the Birmingham Twin Study (Cameron, 1968) amongst more than 500 dichorionic placentae; in each case there was an artery–artery and a vein–vein anastomosis. Both sets of twins were alike in sex and in all the genetic markers tested and it was therefore considered that there was a high probability that they were monozygotic twins.

Whilst vascular communications in dichorionic placentae seem to be rare in man, this is not the case in other species. They are very common in cattle, and also occur frequently in marmoset monkeys (Benirschke, 1970; Hamilton and Poswillo, 1972) and the horse (Vandeplassche, Podliachouk and Beaud, 1970; Jeffcott and Whitwell, 1973), but the effects produced by such a common circulation in dichorionic placentation show great contrasts between species and provide a basis for complex problems, particularly with regard to sex differentiation, which still await solution. When there is such a communicating channel between the twins in utero exchanges of blood elements will be likely to occur: these cannot be identified with regard to an individual fetus if the twins are monozygotic (as was the case in the two pairs in the Birmingham survey), but in other species when the twins are usually DZ, it is possible by blood-grouping and chromosomal techniques, to demonstrate a mixture of genotypes in blood and other tissues. This phenomenon is known as *chimerism* and the individual twin is termed a *chimera* (for discussion of the principles see Ford, 1969; Benirschke, 1970). The associated effects are however somewhat anomalous: in cattle and to a lesser extent in sheep, goats and pigs, the female member of unlike sexed twins is usually sterile and known as a *freemartin*, but this situation is unknown in man and the marmoset monkey. It is presumed that, by analogy with cattle, the mechanism of chimerism in human twins is by the interchange of blood elements through placental anastomoses, but until very recently there has not been an opportunity to observe placental anastomoses and the blood findings in the same case, thus providing absolute proof of causation. However, this has now been provided in a report from Nigeria by Nylander and Osunkoya (1970): these workers describe the placenta from the delivery of a pair of twins of unlike sex. This was thought originally to be monochorionic and an area suggesting vascular anastomosis could be seen on naked eye inspection, but as the placenta had been preserved in formolsaline it was not possible to confirm this by injection studies. The appearance of the fetal surface was somewhat unusual for a monochorionic placenta however and subsequent histological examination showed two layers of chorionic tissue in part of the dividing septum. It was therefore presumed that this had originally been a dichorionic placenta in which the two layers of chorion in the septum had fused and disappeared leaving only traces at the base of the septum. The twins were quite normal on clinical examination after delivery and in particular the genitalia did not show any anomalies. Chromosome studies by Dr. M. K. Lucas at the Galton Laboratory, University College London (personal communication, 1975) showed a mixture of male and female karyotypes in each twin. Specimens of blood were taken at the age of four months. Two lymphocyte cultures were set up from each specimen: 100 cells were examined from each child. In the male twin four cells showed a female karyotype. In the female twin 82 cells showed a male karyotype. Blood groups and other genetic markers were tested at the Blood Transfusion Centre, University of Ibadan, and also by members of the MRC Human Biochemical Genetics Unit at the Galton Laboratory, University College London. At both centres the reaction of the twins' cells with anti-S when compared with the reaction given by the father's cells strongly suggested that both twins possessed a mixture of Ss and ss cells.

There is therefore good circumstantial evidence that blood interchange can take place, though rarely, between twins with dichorionic placentation. Whether the 'twin-transfusion syndrome' is seen amongst such twins is less clear; there are, however, a few reports suggesting that it might. Walker and Turnbull (1955) describe a dichorionic placenta with contrasting territories: one twin was anaemic with many erythroblasts present, and the other twin polycythaemic. There was no report of an anastomosis in the placenta however and the diagnosis of the twin-transfusion syndrome was not considered. Michaels (1967) also reported a dichorionic placenta with pallor and plethora of the maternal surface: one twin was stillborn but the other was quite normal. There were no haematological investigations on the survivor and there are no post-mortem details on the stillborn fetus, which showed moderate maceration. There is no report of any anastomosis, but it was thought that this might have been a case of the transfusion syndrome. It was not thought that the pallor of one half of the placenta was attributable to the intrauterine death of one twin. The other is that described by Allen (1972) in which dichorionic twins respectively had anaemia and polycythaemia. There was marked pallor of one half of the dichorionic placenta (the territory of the anaemic stillborn baby) but no evident arteriovenous anastomoses (injection studies were not carried out). It was however considered that this too was a case of the transfusion syndrome. Whilst, as has been discussed, it is known that vascular communications must exist in this form of placentation, they are very rare and it is quite possible that the findings in some of these cases might have been due to other causes such as feto-maternal haemorrhage, which might, for example, mimic the transfusion syndrome (Strong and Corney, 1967; Gemme and Verri, 1968; Bryan, 1975) in both clinical and placental findings. Alternatively (Walker and Turnbull, 1955) oxygen supplies might not have been uniform for the twins as a result of areas of preferential blood supply on the uterine wall.

HIGHER MULTIPLE BIRTHS

Naturally occurring human multiple births greater than five in number are uncommon; reports of sextuplets and higher multiples have been recorded but many are based on hearsay and are of doubtful authenticity (Mayer, 1952a, 1952b).

The biological principles involved can be well illustrated by reference to

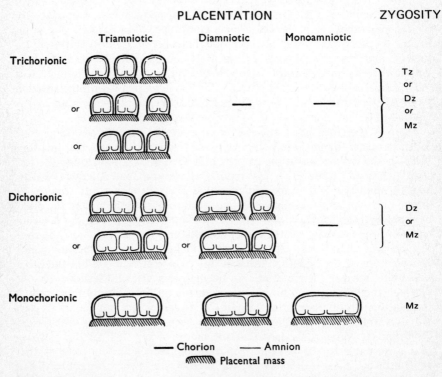

Figure 3.12. Diagram to illustrate placental forms and membrane relationships for the three different types of triplet zygosity. Adapted from Nylander and Corney (1971), by courtesy of the editors, *Annals of Human Genetics* and Cambridge University Press.

triplets, which can originate from (Figure 3.12) three zygotes (TZ), less commonly from two (DZ) and, rarely, from one (MZ). In other words, in the commonest form (TZ triplets), three ova are fertilised by three sperms, but the other two varieties also involve division of a single zygote as in monozygotic twinning. In the case of DZ triplets, initially two ova are fertilised by two sperms, but one of the resulting zygotes then divides and thus the combination is that of a pair of MZ twins and an individual embryo. This of course means that with this type of triplets, as with some of the higher multiple births, the principles of dizygotic and monozygotic twinning are operating

Table 3.8. *Placentation of triplets in hospital samples from the United States, Europe and Nigeria.*

	United States		Germany	England		Nigeria
Placentation	Baltimore (Williams, 1926)	Chicago (Potter & Fuller, 1949)	North Prussia (Steiner, 1935)	Oxford (Corney, Robson and Strong, unpublished data)	Total (Caucasian)	Ibadan
Monochorionic	0	1	1	1	3 (15.8%)	1 (2.5%)
Dichorionic	2[a]	2	3	1	8 (42.1%)	10 (25.0%)
Trichorionic	2	1	2	3	8 (42.1%)	29 (72.5%)
Not known	1	1	1	1	4	4
Total	5	5	7	6	23	44

[a] One set of Negro triplets has been excluded.
Percentages in brackets refer to triplets with known placentation.
From Nylander and Corney (1971), with permission of the editors of *Annals of Human Genetics* and Cambridge University Press.

in the same pregnancy, which might be due to chance, but the mechanism is not at present understood. Those from a single zygote arise because a further division follows the initial cleavage. Multizygotic triplets are commoner than those from a single zygote in populations analysed by the sex-distribution of sets, but because of their infrequent occurrence, similar data on the relative types of quadruplets, quintuplets etc. are much less informative.

Placentation in higher multiple births follows the pattern which has been outlined for twins and again triplets can be used as a model for description (Figure 3.12). As with twin births, monochorionic placentation is the least common (Table 3.8), placentae with two or more chorionic membranes appearing with increasing frequency according to the number of multi-

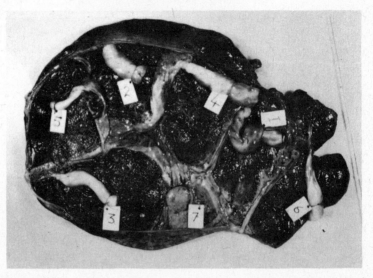

Figure 3.13. Septuplet placenta. From Cameron et al (1969) by courtesy of Dr. A. H. Cameron and the editor, *Journal of Obstetrics and Gynaecology of the British Commonwealth.*

zygotic pregnancies in the population studied. Thus trichorionic placentae are much commoner amongst the Yoruba population in Ibadan, Nigeria, than amongst Caucasian populations in the United States and Europe (Nylander and Corney, 1971). Information with regard to placentation for multiple births higher than three is only available from individual case reports and it is not possible to assess the relative frequencies of the different types. The relevant literature is discussed by Benirschke and Driscoll (1967), Cameron et al (1969), and Boyd and Hamilton (1970).

In recent years the use of gonadotrophins and similar substances for the treatment of infertility has led to an increase in human plural births (Gemzell, Roos and Loeffler, 1968; Hack et al, 1970, 1972). The maximum number so far recorded is apparently nine (Benirschke and Kim, 1973). Such artificially induced multiple pregnancies usually arise from several zygotes as would be expected, because the therapy presumably causes multiple follicles to rupture

Table 3.9. *Result of studies on genetic markers in a set of septuplets.*

	Sex	Blood groups									Placental enzymes		
		ABO	MN	S	C	D	E	c	Kell	Fy^a	PGM_1	PGM_3	Alkaline phosphatase
I	F	A	MM	+	+	+	–	+	–	+	1	1	F
II	M	B	MM	+	+	+	–	+	–	+	1	1	FS
III	F	AB	MM	+	–	–	–	+	–	+	1	2.1	S
IV	F	A	MM	+	–	–	–	+	–	+	1	1	F
V	M	A	MM	+	–	–	–	+	–	+	1	1	FS
VI	F	AB	MM	+	+	+	–	+	–	+	1	1	F
VII	M												

From Cameron et al (1969), with permission of the authors and the editor of *Journal of Obstetrics and Gynaecology of the British Commonwealth*.

thereby releasing several ova. Apprehension that a similar situation might follow the cessation of oral contraceptives as a result of a possible natural 'rebound' of pituitary gonadotrophins seems now to be without foundation as there does not appear to be an increase in multiple pregnancies in this situation (Rice-Wray et al, 1971; Feldmann, Rupek and Tenhaeff, 1971).

An illustration of a multizygotic pregnancy after gonadotrophin therapy is provided by the septuplet pregnancy described by Cameron and his colleagues in 1969. In this case there was a single placental mass (Figure 3.13) in which seven chorionic membranes could be delineated, seven placentae having fused together. Injection studies, as would be expected in this situation, did not reveal any vascular communicating channels between the various placentae. Studies of blood groups (red cell antigens) together with placental enzyme typing and the sex of the babies (Table 3.9) showed that six of the seven infants (it was not possible to determine the zygosity of one) had arisen from separate zygotes. A similar situation was found amongst the sextuplets described by Lachelin et al (1972), all of which had individual chorionic sacs, and genetic markers showed differences between the five on whom such studies were possible.

Other recent reports of higher multiple births, the majority of which followed therapy for infertility, include octuplets (Prokop and Herrmann, 1973). Septuplets were described by Turksoy and his colleagues in 1967 and more recently an interesting set which included two anencephalic infants was described by Burnell (1974), though there are no details of placentation or zygosity. Quintuplets have been reported in recent years by Jewelwicz et al (1972). The set of quadruplets described by Atlay and Pennington (1971) was very unusual as it consisted of dichorionic and monoamniotic twins. Two other descriptions of quadruplets include data on zygosity; those from Mayr, Pausch and Mickerts (1969) originated from four zygotes and a naturally occurring set from Nigeria very exceptionally consisted of two pairs of monochorionic twins (Nylander and Corney, 1971).

CHAPTER 4

The Causation of Twinning

P. P. S. NYLANDER

The aetiology of twinning has been the subject of much investigation for several years and various writers have discussed the hereditary and other factors which may be responsible for monozygotic and dizygotic twinning.

HEREDITARY FACTORS

MONOZYGOTIC TWINNING

Although a few authors like Davenport (1920) and Fisher (1928) believed that monozygotic twinning is determined by heredity on the paternal as well as maternal side, it is now generally accepted that this type of twinning is not influenced by heredity. The fact that the monozygotic twinning rate in different races is fairly constant in spite of obviously different genetic characteristics in these populations is in itself very suggestive that monozygotic twinning is not under hereditary control. Weinberg (1902, 1909) showed that the twinning rate in female relatives of mothers of monozygotic twins (estimated by his method, 1902) was approximately the same as that in the general population, while female relatives of mothers of unlike-sexed (i.e., dizygotic) twins had a twinning rate which was about twice that in the general population. He therefore concluded that monozygotic twinning was not inherited. Other investigations (Greulich, 1934; Bulmer, 1960) have confirmed this finding.

It therefore appears that monozygotic twinning is a chance phenomenon and is not under hereditary control. Some of the contradictory results obtained from investigations by earlier workers were probably due to biased data.

DIZYGOTIC TWINNING

Weinberg (1909), Greulich (1934), Dahlberg (1952), Bulmer (1958), and Wyshak and White (1965) have shown that there is a considerable increase in the repeat frequency of twinning for dizygotic twinning but not for mono-zygotic twinning, i.e., a woman who has had monozygotic twins is not any more likely to have twins than other women in the general population, whereas a mother of dizygotic twins has a much higher tendency to twinning than other women in the general population. This finding does not, of course, indicate whether the greater propensity to dizygotic twinning in some women is due to genetic or environmental causes. Further investigations have, how-ever, been done by these and other authors to elucidate the cause of this proneness to dizygotic twinning in some women. The findings have shown lack of agreement among these investigators. There are those like Davenport (1920, 1927), Curtius (1928), Eckert (1928), Meyer (1932) and Greulich (1934) who concluded that dizygotic twinning was inherited from both the maternal and paternal side. For example, Greulich in his study of twinning rates among the parents and siblings of 495 pairs of twins, concluded that the capacity to produce dizygotic twins was at least as pronounced on the father's side as on the mother's side. However, as Bulmer (1970) has pointed out, it is likely that there was bias in Greulich's data due to under-reporting of singletons on the paternal side. This would have the effect of inflating the corresponding twinning rate. This tendency to under-reporting of singleton births on the paternal side has been amply illustrated by data collected by Bulmer (1960) in his own study. He found high twinning rates (due to under-reporting of singletons) among the father's brothers and sisters. However, after correcting for this under-reporting, the adjusted rates were found to be only slightly above the expected rates. It is likely that this source of bias is responsible for the findings of other investigators who have found that dizygotic twinning is influenced by the genotype of the father.

Isolated cases are, however, described from time to time which are very suggestive that the paternal genotype influences dizygotic twinning. Browne (1946) in his book on ante-natal and post-natal care, has quoted cases in which each of the two spouses of a particular husband had had multiple births at every maternity. For example, the case of a Russian peasant is cited, who had 64 children by his two wives, the first wife having had quadruplets four times, triplets seven times, twins six times and the second wife, triplets once and twins six times. Another case quoted was that of a husband whose wife had 21 children in seven successive pregnancies and whose servant-maid, having been seduced by him, had triplets. Further evidence of this nature is given by Oettle (1953) who had described a pedigree in which certain males appeared to have been able to induce a high incidence of multiple births. He was unfortunately unable to confirm the details of the family tree which was obtained from only one person.

Those who have advocated that the paternal genotype influences dizygotic twinning have adduced various theories for the mechanism which accounts for this astonishing finding. Guttmacher (1939b) suggested that in some cases the sperms might have the capacity to fertilise polar bodies. This advocates the existence of a third type of twinning, which has not been proved. Other authors, e.g., Davenport (1920), Lenz (1933), have suggested that poly-ovulation occurs more commonly than is believed and that at fertilisation, one of the following may happen:

1. Only one of the two or more ova shed may be fertilised because of incapacity of the sperms to fertilise more than one egg, or because of limited duration of fertility in the sperms, or the formation of some substances which prevent the fertilisation of other ova.

2. More than one ovum may be fertilised, and all but one may fail to complete their development due to lethal factors in the sperms. The sperms of fathers of dizygotic twins are supposed to be more active, numerous, without lethal factors and with longer duration of fertility, so that more ova are fertilised and more fertilised ova complete their development. Attractive as this theory is, there is however no evidence that some sperms have inherited capacity to fertilise ova more than other sperms, nor have any substances which inhibit fertilisation been isolated from spermatozoa.

Investigators who have advocated that the tendency to dizygotic twinning is inherited only on the maternal side include Weinberg (1909), Danforth (1916), Bonnevie (1919), Wehefritz (1925), Dahlberg (1926), Lenz (1933), Bulmer (1960) and White and Wyshak (1964). Reference to Weinberg's and Bulmer's findings was made previously. Both investigators found an increased twinning rate in female relatives of mothers of twins. White and Wyshak (1964) using family records from the Mormon Church of Salt Lake City found that women who were themselves dizygotic twins and the female sibs of such women had twinning rates which were much higher than that in the general population, whereas men who were themselves dizygotic twins and their male siblings had twinning rates which were not higher than that in the general population. For example, they found that the twinning rate in the offspring of 365 women who were themselves dizygotic twins was 17.1 per 1000 maternities—significantly higher than that for the general population (11.6 per 1000 maternities). In contrast the twinning rate in the offspring of 586 males who were themselves dizygotic twins was only 7.9 per 1000 maternities. They therefore concluded that the genotype of the mother affected the twinning rate but that of the father did not. Further evidence in support of this finding has come from Morton (1962) who, studying children of inter-racial marriages in Hawaii, found that the frequency of dizygotic twinning depended on the mother's race and was independent of the father's race.

Populations in tropical Africa, many of which have high twinning rates with high proportions of dizygotic twins, are obviously suitable fields in which hereditary tendency in dizygotic twins can be investigated. Furthermore, the widespread practice of polygyny in many such populations provides a good opportunity for investigating paternal influence on dizygotic twinning. Such an investigation was carried out recently in Ibadan, Western Nigeria (Nylander, 1970c). An added advantage of conducting the study in this population is the prominence which is given to twin births in the community (for example, special names are given to twins and special ceremonies performed for them). This ensured that a history of twinning in the family was not missed and also stimulated interest in studies in the factor of inheritance in twinning.

Among 18 737 deliveries in two hospitals in Ibadan there were 977 twin maternities. Every mother was interrogated immediately after delivery to

find out whether she or her husband was a twin or had had twins previously
(including those delivered by the husband's other wives), and whether she or
her husband had twin siblings. Obstetric data, including maternal age and
parity, were collected for each patient, as mentioned previously, and zygosity
of the newborn twins was determined by sex, placentation, blood groups,
placental enzymes, haemoglobin types, and G6PD electrophoretic studies.

In this population about 92 per cent of twins at birth are dizygotic
(Nylander, 1969). Since there is a much higher perinatal and infant mortality
among monozygotic twins, the proportion of dizygotic twins in the adult
population is likely to be much higher than 92 per cent. The data in this
investigation, therefore, relate mainly to dizygotic twinning.

Table 4.1 has been divided into two parts: Part A shows data relating to
the women themselves and their husbands, Part B shows data relating to the
women and their parents.

Table 4.1. *Types of women and proportion who delivered twins and singletons, in Ibadan.*

Types of women	Those who delivered twins	Those who delivered singletons
Part A		
(1) Women who are themselves twins	72 (7.4%)	1418 (8.0%)
(2) Women who have had twins previously	199 (20.4%)	1973 (11.1%)
(3) Women whose husbands are themselves twins	61 (6.2%)	1250 (7.0%)
(4) Women whose husbands have had twins	258 (26.4%)	3101 (17.5%)
(5) Women whose husbands have had twins by other wives	59 (6.0%)	1128 (6.4%)
Part B		
(1) Women whose mothers are themselves twins	41 (4.2%)	714 (4.0%)
(2) Women whose mothers have had twins	221 (22.6%)	2806 (15.8%)
(3) Women whose fathers are themselves twins	33 (3.4%)	444 (2.5%)
(4) Women whose fathers have had twins	247 (25.3%)	3213 (18.1%)
(5) Women whose fathers have had twins by other wives	26 (2.7%)	407 (2.3%)

Figures in parenthesis indicate the percentage of the total number of maternities of those
who delivered twins (977) or those who delivered singletons (17 760).

In Table 4.1A, five types of woman have been described, namely (1) those
who are themselves twins; (2) those who have had twins previously; (3) those
whose husbands are themselves twins; (4) those whose husbands have had
twins (i.e., by other wives as well); (5) those whose husbands have had twins
by other wives—data for this fifth category of patients are derived by
subtracting the figures for patients who have had twins previously from those
for patients whose husbands have had twins (by other wives as well). All the
patients have been divided into two groups, depending on whether they
delivered twins or singletons, and the proportion of each type of patient out
of the total number of patients in each group has been shown. It will be seen
that the proportion of women who are themselves twins is approximately the
same in the 'twin' and 'singleton' groups of women. The findings are similar
for women who have had twins previously, and women whose husbands have

had twins previously (by other wives as well), namely that the values are much higher in the 'twin' group of patients.

The data have been expressed as rates per thousand maternities in Table 4.2A. Women who are themselves twins and those who are not have approximately the same twinning rates. Women whose husbands are themselves twins and those whose husbands are not also have similar twinning rates.

Table 4.2. *Twinning rates in different types of women.*

Types of women	Twinning rate per 1000 maternities	Types of women	Twinning rate per 1000 maternities
Part A			
(1) Women who are themselves twins	48.3	Women who are not twins	52.5
(2) Women who have had twins previously	91.6	Women who have not had twins previously	47.0
(3) Women whose husbands are themselves twins	46.5	Women whose husbands are not twins	52.6
(4) Women whose husbands have had twins	76.8	Women whose husbands have not had twins	46.8
(5) Women whose husbands have had twins by other wives	49.7	Women whose husbands have not had twins by other wives	52.3
Part B			
(1) Women whose mothers are themselves twins	54.3	Women whose mothers are not twins	52.1
(2) Women whose mothers have had twins	73.0	Women whose mothers have not had twins	48.1
(3) Women whose fathers are themselves twins	69.2	Women whose fathers are not twins	51.7
(4) Women whose fathers have had twins	71.4	Women whose fathers have not had twins	47.8
(5) Women whose fathers have had twins by other wives	60.0	Women whose fathers have not had twins by other wives	52.0

However, women who have had twins previously have a twinning rate about twice that of their counterparts who have not. The twinning rate among women whose husbands have had twins by other wives is about the same as that among women whose husbands have not. This indicates that the husbands have not contributed to the twinning tendency.

Since twinning rates are influenced by maternal age and parity, the data for the two groups of women in Table 4.2A—those who have had twins previously and those who have not—have been analysed by maternal age and parity. In each age and parity group, women who have had twins previously are found to have much higher twinning rates than those who have not. The figures for women in the second parity group are shown in Table 4.3 to illustrate this point. It will be seen from this table that the twinning rates in both groups of women rise up to a peak at the age of 30 to 34 years but the rates in the first group are always much higher than those in the second group.

Table 4.3. *Twinning rates (‰ maternities) in patients who have had two previous deliveries analysed by maternal age.*

	Maternal age groups				
	15–19	20–24	25–29	30–34	35–39
Patients who have had twins previously	71.4	74.1	107.5	111.1	76.9
Patients who have not had twins previously	25.6	48.6	62.0	68.0	30.6
Total no. of patients	53	1028	1811	614	111

In Table 4.2B five other categories of women are described, namely: (1) women whose mothers are themselves twins; (2) women whose mothers have had twins (i.e., women who have twin siblings or are themselves a twin; (3) women whose fathers are themselves twins; (4) women whose fathers have had twins (by all wives); (5) women whose fathers have had twins by other wives—data for this fifth category of women have been derived in the same way as in Table 4.1A (i.e., by subtracting data from women of type 2 from data for those of type 4).

The women whose mothers are themselves twins have a twinning rate which is similar to that for women whose mothers are not twins (Table 4.2B). But women whose mothers have had twins (i.e., women who are either themselves twins or who have twin siblings) have a twinning rate which is significantly higher than women whose mothers have not had twins (i.e., women who are neither twins themselves nor have they twin siblings). Also women whose fathers are themselves twins have a twinning rate which *appears* to be higher than that for women whose fathers are not twins, but the difference between the two rates is not significant. The twinning rate in women whose fathers have had twins (71.4/1000 maternities) is significantly higher than that in women whose fathers have not had twins but this is because this group includes data for women whose mothers have had twins previously, who have a high twinning rate, since the twinning rate in women whose fathers had twins by other wives is not significantly higher than that in women whose fathers have not had twins by other wives.

The analysis of data for all the ten categories of women, therefore, shows that only two groups of women have twinning rates which are significantly higher than that in the general population, namely: (1) women who have had twins previously; (2) women whose mothers have had twins. Other groups of women, in particular those who are themselves twins and those whose mothers are themselves twins, have twin rates which are similar to that in the general population.

The Ibadan study has helped to *indicate* whether genetic or environmental factors play the greater role in the aetiology of dizygotic twinning *in that population*.

Firstly, the following findings—(a) women whose husbands are themselves twins have similar twinning rates to women whose husbands are not twins; (b) women whose husbands have had twins by other wives have similar twinning rates to women whose husbands have not had twins by other wives; (c) women whose fathers are twins have a twinning rate not significantly higher than that for women whose fathers are not twins; and (d) women whose fathers have had twins by other wives have similar twinning rates to women whose fathers have not had twins by other wives—suggest that fathers do not contribute to the twinning tendency. This finding is in agreement with that of Morton (1962) and White and Wyshak (1964).

Secondly, the finding that women who have had twins previously have a twinning rate which is almost twice that in women who have not had twins is also in agreement with that in many other investigations in Caucasian populations (White and Wyshak, 1964 etc.). The high twinning tendency in this group of women could be due to genetic or environmental factors.

Thirdly, the findings that (a) women who are themselves twins are not any more likely to twinning than women who are not themselves twins, and that (b) women whose mothers are themselves twins are not any more likely to have twins than women whose mothers are not twins, are contrary to the findings in many other investigations in Caucasian populations (e.g., Bulmer, 1960; White and Wyshak, 1964). These findings (in the Ibadan population) are difficult to reconcile with the theory of genetic determination of twinning.

There is thus evidence from the Ibadan and other studies that dizygotic twinning is not inherited on the paternal side. The findings in most studies indicate that this type of twinning is influenced only by the genotype of the mother. The exact nature of the inheritance is still in doubt. Many views have been expressed—sex-limited recessive trait (Wehefritz, 1925), Mendelian recessive (Weinberg, 1909; Curtius, 1928; Bulmer, 1970, etc.). McArthur (1952) in her investigation using records of attendances at antenatal clinics has suggested that maternal recessive genes are responsible, but so far no one theory has been found entirely satisfactory.

OTHER CAUSES OF TWINNING

MONOZYGOTIC TWINNING

It has been shown that there is very little evidence that hereditary factors play a part in monozygotic twinning. The monozygotic twinning rate varies so little under so many varying conditions that one is led to believe that this type of twinning is due to chance. It is, however, likely that the remarkably consistent frequency of this type of twinning is a reflection of the constancy of the environment in the human Fallopian tubes and uterus, which protects the fertilised egg from external influences at the time when development begins. It is probable, therefore, that the cause of this type of twinning is to be found in slight temporary changes which may occur in the environment of the developing embryo during its early stages.

Some investigations (Mall, 1908; Patterson, 1913; Stockard, 1921; Arey, 1922; Sturkie, 1946) have suggested that such a change might be caused by lack of oxygen and nutrition due to delay in implantation of the developing egg, and that this deficiency could cause developmental arrest which would in turn result in abnormal development or division of the embryo when growth resumed. In favour of this theory is the apparent association of delay in implantation and developmental arrest (or retardation of development, produced experimentally) (Loeb, 1909) with polyembryony in certain animal species—the armadillo and sea-urchin. However, similar delay in implantation and developmental arrest in other animal species—roe-deer and badgers —is not associated with monozygotic twinning (Bischoff, 1854; Hamlett, 1933). Another finding which appeared to support this theory was the claim by Arey (1922) that monochorionic placentation (which is invariably associated with monozygotic twins) occurred far more frequently in tubal than in uterine pregnancies. He suggested that oxygen lack and impaired blood supply which was more likely to be associated with the delay in implantation and ectopic gestation was responsible for the increased frequency of monozygotic twinning. However, as Bulmer (1970) pointed out, Arey did not include bilateral tubal pregnancies in his investigation, which was therefore biased in favour of monozygotic twins since some dizygotic twins (from bilateral tubal pregnancies) would have been omitted, while all the monozygotic ones would be included.

Many authors, like Stockard, have also drawn attention to the finding that oxygen lack and developmental arrest would cause congenital malformation or monozygotic twinning in some animal species depending on the stage of development at which the arrest occurred. This theory, therefore, regards monozygotic twinning as a form of abnormal development similar in aetiology to congenital malformation. Another point of similarity between monozygotic twinning and congenital malformation is in their relation to maternal age. The incidence of congenital malformation increases with maternal age. Monozygotic twinning, though remarkably constant under a wide range of conditions, nevertheless shows a slight increase with maternal age. A further point of similarity is the finding that the incidence of congenital malformation is much higher in monozygotic twinning than in dizygotic twinning.

Other theories which have been proposed regarding the cause of monozygotic twinning include defects in the sperm or ovum (Broman, 1902; Kaestner, 1912) and weakness of the zona pellucida which is said to allow early separation of the cells of the segmenting ovum. There is, however, very little evidence to support these views. The cause of monozygotic twinning in man is still obscure and most of the evidence which has been obtained so far is only suggestive that monozygotic twinning, like congenital malformations, may be associated with developmental arrest due to oxygen lack.

DIZYGOTIC TWINNING

Dizygotic twinning occurs from the fertilisation of two ova shed at ovulation. In spite of extensive research the exact mechanism responsible for this double ovulation is not clearly understood, but a consideration of the biological processes leading to ovulation may indicate some of the possible factors. At the beginning of the menstrual cycle, several Graafian follicles (in both ovaries), influenced by follicle stimulating hormone (FSH) secreted by the anterior pituitary, begin to mature. Development of the follicles continues during the first half of the menstrual cycle as the level of FSH in the blood increases. The developing follicles themselves secrete oestrogens which stimulate growth of the lining of the uterus (endometrium). Almost always, one follicle outstrips the others in development and it is this follicle that ruptures at ovulation under the influence of a surge of luteinising hormone (LH) and FSH secreted by the anterior pituitary. After ovulation the level of FSH falls and atresia continues in the other follicles which have not ovulated. (The foregoing is a simplified account which is generally accepted, although different endocrinologists vary in their opinions regarding the minute details.) The reason why many of the follicles fail to reach maturity and ovulate is obscure. It is possible that their development is in some ways inhibited by the 'more mature' follicles or that each follicle varies in its sensitivity and reaction to FSH. The mechanism responsible for two follicles ovulating on certain occasions and the factors determining the ovary from which such ovulation occurs, are also obscure. A possibility is that the different follicles develop at different rates, but if at the time of the LH and FSH surge two follicles in either or both ovaries happen to have reached *precisely* the same point of maturity physiologically, then both are ovulated. Once ovulation has occurred, the fall in the serum FSH level would reduce further ovarian stimulation so that no further development would occur in the other follicles. This view, however, is conjectural and there is as yet no evidence to support it.

A rise in the dizygotic twinning rate is likely to be due to an increase in the frequency of double ovulation. It has been suggested that usually at double ovulation, only one of the ova is fertilised. The second ovum may not be fertilised because of incapacity of the sperms or some other factor. If such is the case any factors which increase the probability of the fertilisation of two ova will cause an increase in the dizygotic twinning rate. Furthermore, it is believed by some that only a proportion of the double embryos occurring from fertilisation at double ovulation result in twin births; in the others, one or both embryos have perished and been absorbed during the early months of pregnancy. If this is so, any factors causing a decrease in the mortality rate of such embryos will result in increasing the dizygotic twinning rate. There is, however, very little evidence that an increase in the rate of fertilisation of two ova or a decrease in the mortality rate of twin embryos, are responsible for variation in dizygotic twinning rate. On the contrary there is plenty of evidence to indicate that a high dizygotic twinning frequency can be caused by increased multiple ovulation. The use of exogenous gonadotrophins, clomiphene or similar drugs in the treatment of infertile women has been shown to cause a rise in serum FSH and induce multiple ovulation, resulting in multiple births in a high proportion of cases (Gemzell and Roos, 1966; Jacobson et al, 1968), much higher than expected from the incidence of multiple births in the general population. The rise in urinary gonadotrophins with advancing maternal age reported by Albert et al (1956) has been regarded as further evidence that the frequency of multiple ovulation is controlled by the level of pituitary gonadotrophin in the blood. Loraine (1963) on the other hand found that urinary pituitary gonadotrophin levels did not rise with maternal age. These tests were carried out in urine using bio-assay methods and the results have not been substantiated by the more recent and accurate methods of estimation of gonadotrophin levels in serum or plasma. Furthermore, since twinning rates also increase with parity it would be expected that gonadotrophin levels should also increase with parity, if this is the mechanism by which maternal age and parity influence the incidence of twinning. But this has also not been substantiated by accurate methods of estimation of serum gonadotrophins. Obviously more research is needed in this field using modern methods of assay.

It has been suggested that anatomical and functional differences in the pituitary may explain the variation of twinning rates with maternal age, parity and race (Milham, 1964). This suggestion has been criticised (Eriksson, 1964) on the grounds that many factors (including a high rate of embryonic deaths, environmental and genetic factors) influence the dizygotic twinning rate and the hypophysis (and hypothalamus) may be only one. If a high rate of embryonic death is an important factor in determining variation in twinning rate one would expect greater variation in monozygotic twinning rates, since embryonic deaths are more likely to occur in monozygotic twins (most of which share one placenta). Instead, the monozygotic twinning rate is remarkably constant. Furthermore, it is possible that environmental and genetic factors may exert their influence on dizygotic twinning by causing alteration in the function of the anterior pituitary and the level of gonadotrophins.

A recent study (Nylander, 1973) of serum gonadotrophin levels in Ibadan women appears to lend some support to the hypothesis that women who are twin-prone have higher levels of serum gonadotrophin. Fifteen mothers participated in the study—six who had delivered only singleton babies, seven who had each delivered one set of twins and two who had delivered two sets of twins. It has been found that the mean daily serum concentration of FSH four days before and after the FSH peak was higher in the women who had delivered twins than in those who had delivered singletons. Furthermore, the women who had delivered two sets of twins had the highest mean FSH concentration. There did not appear to be any association of twinning with serum LH levels. Although the number of mothers investigated was too small to show statistically significant differences, the findings were suggestive that there is an association of twinning with serum FSH levels.

Further investigations, for example large studies of pituitary gonadotrophin levels in different populations, are indicated to determine the role of environmental and genetic factors in the function of the anterior pituitary, level of gonadotrophins and dizygotic twinning.

CHAPTER 5

Frequency of Multiple Births

P. P. S. NYLANDER

TWINNING RATES

The twinning rates in different parts of the world may be studied by considering three main groups of populations:

1. Those with relatively high twinning rates, e.g. populations in Africa (Table 5.1).
2. Those with relatively low twinning rates, e.g. populations in the Far East (Table 5.2).
3. Those with twinning rates which are intermediate, e.g. Europe, U.S.A., India and Pakistan (Table 5.3).

In populations in Europe and the United States, the relevant data have usually been collected from maternal birth statistics, but in most of the other countries (in Africa and Asia) the source of the data has been mostly from hospital or midwives' records and the size of some samples has been small. Monozygotic and dizygotic twinning rates in these studies have been calculated by Weinberg's method. What has come to be known as 'Weinberg's method' for estimating the numbers of dizygotic and monozygotic twin pairs in a population was first stated by him in 1901 and published in the following year. In fact the same approach had been put forward by Bertillon in 1874, but was not apparently acceptable to contemporary opinion. The method uses the distribution of the numbers of like and unlike-sexed pairs in a population to estimate the numbers of dizygotic and monozygotic pairs. It is based on the fact that, as the sex of each member of a dizygotic pair is determined independently, there will therefore be equal numbers of pairs of like and unlike sex. In other words if the number of pairs of different sex in a population is doubled, this will represent the number of dizygotic pairs. This

Table 5.1. *Rates of twinning in Africa.*

Author	Date of investigation	Place in Africa	Population	Incidence of twins/1000 births			Other information
				Total	Dizygous	Mono-zygous	
Bulmer (1960)	1954–58	Gambia	Bathurst, birth statistics	16.6	9.9	6.7	Based on only 57 twins
	No date	Nigeria	Ibadan, hospital statistics	44.9	39.9	5.0	603 twins
	No date	S. Rhodesia	Salisbury ,, ,,	28.9	26.6	2.3	100 twins
	No date	Congo	Leopoldville ,, ,,	21.8	18.7	3.1	500 twins
			Elisabethville ,, ,,	16.9	13.3	3.6	270 twins
Jeffreys (1953)		Transvaal	Swazi	28	24	4	28 twins
		Natal	Zulu	28	21	7	116 twins
Bulmer (1960)		Zululand	Zulu	22	21	1	92 twins
Jeffreys (1953)		N. Transvaal	Shangaan	41	32	9	41 twins
		N. Transvaal	Xosa	27	27	0	29 twins
		Bechuanaland	Tswana	18	10	8	87 twins
Bulmer (1960)		Johannesburg		20	16	4	710 twins
		Johannesburg		27	22	5	290 twins
Jeffreys (1953)		Durban		23	21	2	66 twins
Stevenson et al (1966)		Pretoria		20	17	3	197 twins
Ross (1952)		Cape Town	'Cape coloured'	13	5	8	40 twins
Bulmer (1960)		S. Rhodesia	Mashona	29	27	2	100 twins
		Leopoldville		22	19	3	500 twins
		Elisabethville		17	13	4	270 twins
Roberts and Tanner (1963)		Tanganyika	Hangaza	24	20	4	39 twins
Jeffreys (1953)		Br. Camerons	Banso	16	13	3	72 twins
Cox (1963)		E. Nigeria	Ibo	33	23	10	109 twins
Jeffreys (1953)		S. Nigeria	Ibo	27	22	5	90 twins
Bulmer (1960)		Ibadan, Nigeria	Yoruba	45	40	5	603 twins
Knox and Morley (1960)		Ilesha, W. Nigeria	Yoruba	54	49	5	158 twins
Nylander (1969)		Igbo-Ora, W. Nigeria	Yoruba	46	42	4	177 twins
Bulmer (1960)		Gambia		17	10	7	57 twins

Data presented in Tables 5.1, 5.2 and 5.3 are adapted from tables in Hytten and Leitch (1964) and Bulmer (1970).

Table 5.2. *Rates of twinning in Asia.*

Author	Date of investigation	Place in Far East	Population	Incidence of twins/1000 births			Other information
				Total	Dizygous	Mono-zygous	
Millis (1959)	1950–53	Singapore	Poor Chinese in hospital	10.9	4.2	6.7	
Komai and Fukuoka (1936)	1926–31	Japan	Midwives' records from Osaka Honshu Kyushu	5.6 6.8 7.1	2.7 2.9 2.6	2.9 3.9 4.5	Authors say data from Korea and Formosa similar
Morton (1955)	post–1945 no detail	Japan	Nagasaki and Hiroshima; total birth statistics	4.3	1.3	3.0	
Kandror (1961)	1944–46 1946–50	U.S.S.R	Arctic region	7.7	—	—	9 sets of twins in 1181 births

of course is less than the total number of twins in the population and the difference represents the number of monozygotic pairs. Thus:

(No. of monozygotic pairs) = (Total No. of pairs) − 2 (No. of pairs of unlike sex)

Discrepancies such as the slightly higher number of male births do not appear to invalidate the method (Bulmer, 1970).

The twinning rate in European countries and the United States is generally between about 10 and 15 per 1000 maternities. The dizygotic twinning rate varies between 7 and 11 per 1000 maternities, but the monozygotic rate is fairly constant between 3 and 4 per 1000 maternities. The incidence in the Negroes in the United States—14.9 per 1000 maternities—is higher than that of the Caucasians—10.6 per 1000 maternities (Shipley et al, 1967), but it is no higher than that seen in some Caucasian populations, for example, Rumania —15.6 per 1000 maternities (Bulmer, 1960). The twinning rates in India and Pakistan, apart from that for Lahore, appear on the whole to be similar to those in Europe, the rates varying from 9 per 1000 maternities in Baroda to 17 per 1000 maternities in Patna (Bulmer, 1970). The rates are based on hospital data and are therefore subject to varying degrees of bias. (The incidence of 23 per 1000 reported for Lahore is probably very inflated because of a high degree of such bias.) The dizygotic twinning rates vary from 7 to 11 per 1000 and the monozygotic twinning rates from 3 to 6 per 1000. This variation in the dizygotic twinning rate is likely to be a reflection of the varying degrees of hospital selection in the data.

The twinning rates in the African Negroes are higher, and in some cases several times higher, than those in populations in Europe and the United States. The rates vary from 16 per 1000 in the Gambia to 45 per 1000 in Nigeria (Bulmer, 1960; Nylander, 1967), the dizygotic twinning rates varying from 10 to 40 per 1000 maternities and the monozygotic rates from 3 to 6 per 1000 maternities. Here again, the data have been collected from hospital records and the variation in monozygotic rates is probably due to hospital bias.

The twinning rates in Asia (i.e., among the Japanese, Chinese, Koreans, etc.) are generally much lower than those in Europe and the U.S.A. If the pre-war birth statistics for the Japanese and Chinese are omitted since they are believed to be inaccurate due to under-reporting, reported figures from hospital records vary from 6 per 1000 maternities in Japan (Komai and Fukuoka, 1936) to 14 per 1000 maternities in Korea (Kang and Cho, 1962). The variation in the dizygotic twinning rate is from 2 to 8 per 1000 maternities and in monozygotic rate from 3 to 7 per 1000 maternities. Some of the data have been obtained from hospital records and the twinning rates in these cases are likely to be inflated. This probably also accounts for the varying monozygotic twinning rates in these populations.

Since many of the twinning rates have been obtained from hospital records, it is important to consider how representative rates obtained from such sources are of the incidence in the general population. Firstly there is a tendency for twinning rates in most hospitals to be inflated because of preferential admission of twin maternities (on account of the higher risk of complications). In hospitals which deliver only normal maternities, the incidence of twinning will be lower than that in the general population (Nylander, 1969). Secondly the age and parity distribution in hospital maternities may be very different from that in the general population, especially in developing countries. This may result from (1) hospital practice of preferential booking of one group of patients (e.g., young primigravida or grand multiparous patients), or (2) from self-selection due to certain groups of patients, e.g. multigravida preferring to be confined at home, or (3) migration of groups of people (e.g., young women in search of employment) into large cities where maternity hospitals are situated (Nylander, 1970d). This bias relating to age and parity structure of the hospital sample may affect not only the overall twinning rate but also the proportion of monozygotic and dizygotic twins in the sample, since dizygotic twinning rates vary with maternal age and parity. For these reasons great care has to be taken in interpreting twinning rates derived from hospital data.

It is however possible to use selected cases from these hospital data to derive the approximate twinning rate in the general population. This can be done in two ways:

ANALYSIS OF BOOKED PATIENTS ONLY

Booked patients in a hospital are those who have previously had antenatal care in that hospital. The other group of delivered mothers are those who have come to hospital for delivery on account of some complication in labour. In many hospitals it is this latter group that is largely responsible for inflating the twinning rate, since complications are more common with twin deliveries. Therefore, if the twinning rate is calculated in booked patients only in some hospitals, an incidence similar to that in the general population may be obtained (Nylander, 1969).

In many hospitals, however, selection factors can also occur even in booked patients such as:

1. The booking of patients with uncomplicated twin pregnancies in preference to other pregnant patients.
2. The booking of patients because of complications during pregnancy. A disproportionately large number of patients with twin pregnancy are found in this group of patients since antenatal complications such as hydramnios and pre-eclampsia occur more frequently in patients with twin pregnancies. The effect of this factor is to increase the twinning rate in hospital populations.
3. The relatively high proportion of young primigravidae who register for antenatal care in some hospitals. The incidence of twinning is lower in this group of patients.

In some hospitals the last two factors tend to cancel each other out, thereby giving a twinning rate close to that in the general community.

ANALYSIS OF CASES BOOKED EARLY IN PREGNANCY

The bias which may occur in booked patients in some hospitals may be

Table 5.3. *Rates of twinning in Europe, U.S.A., India and Pakistan.*

Author	Date of investigation	Place	Population	Incidence of twins/1000 births			Other information
				Total	Dizygous	Mono-zygous	
Bulmer (1960)		*Europe*					
	1951–53	Spain	National birth statistics	9.1	5.9	3.2	Standardised for maternal age
	1955–56	Portugal	,,	10.1	6.5	3.6	
	1946–51	France	,,	10.8	7.1	3.7	
	1950	Belgium	,,	10.9	7.3	3.6	
	1952–56	Austria	,,	10.9	7.5	3.4	
	1901–53	Luxembourg	,,	11.4	7.9	3.5	
	1950–55	West Germany	,,	11.5	8.2	3.3	
	1930–32	Lithuania	,,	11.5	—	—	
	1935–41	Hungary	,,	11.6	—	—	
	1931–32	Poland	,,	11.7	—	—	
	1946–55	Sweden	,,	11.7	8.6	3.2	
	1943–48	Switzerland	,,	11.7	8.1	3.6	
	1946–55	Holland	,,	11.9	8.1	3.7	
	1935–39	Bulgaria	,,	11.9	—	—	
	1946–54	Norway	,,	12.1	8.3	3.8	
	1949–55	Italy	,,	12.3	8.6	3.7	
	1950–55	East Germany	,,	12.4	9.1	3.3	
	1955	Yugoslavia	,,	12.6	—	—	
	1931–33	Czechoslovakia	,,	13.2	9.8	3.4	
	1931–38	Greece	,,	13.8	10.9	2.9	
	1946–55	Denmark	,,	14.2	—	—	
	1935–37	Finland	,,	14.6	—	—	
	1935–37	Estonia	,,	15.1	—	—	
	1936–38	Rumania	,,	15.6	—	—	
	1935–38	Latvia	,,	16.3	—	—	
Registrar-General (1958)	1938–56	England and Wales	National birth statistics	12.3	8.8	3.5	
Karn (1952)	1927–48	London	University College Hospital	16.6	10.9	5.7	

Source	Date	Place	Type of statistics				Notes
Anderson (1956)	1938–52	Aberdeen	Maternity hospital	15.2	—	—	Stillbirths before the 28th week of pregnancy excluded
	1939–52	Scotland	National birth statistics	13.9	—	—	
Nylander (1970b)	1950–65	Aberdeen	Maternity hospital	12.5	8.2	4.3	
Bulmer (1958)	1938	*United States* U.S.A.	White population statistics	11.3	7.1	4.2	Figures adjusted from those published by Enders and Stern (1948)[a]
			Negro	15.8	11.1	4.7	
Statistical Bulletin of the Metropolitan Life Insurance Co. (1960)	1951–57	U.S.A.	White population statistics	10.1	—	—	At least one twin surviving
			Negro	13.4	—	—	
Bulmer (1970)		*India and Pakistan* Ahmedabad	Hospital statistics	12.9	7.6	5.3	225 twins
		Bangalore	,,	10.2	7.3	2.9	493 twins
		Baroda	,,	8.7	6.2	2.5	118 twins
		Bombay	,,	11.1	6.8	4.3	1643 twins
		Bombay	,,	12.2	7.2	5.0	490 twins
Stevenson et al (1966)		Calcutta	,,	11.4	8.1	3.3	876 twins
Bulmer (1970)		Calcutta	,,	13.8	11.0	2.8	268 twins
Stevenson et al (1966)		Dibrugarh	,,	10.5	7.0	3.5	105 twins
Bulmer (1970)		Hyderabad	,,	12.9	7.9	5.0	258 twins
		Lahore	,,	23.3	15.5	7.8	108 twins
		Lucknow	,,	13.2	8.0	5.2	109 twins
		Nagpur	,	17.5	11.1	6.4	164 twins
		Patna	,,	17.4	11.2	6.2	115 twins
		Trivandrum	,,	16.9	9.0	7.9	278 twins
		Visakhapatnam	,,	13.2	8.5	4.7	361 twins

[a] Figures were originally published by Enders, T. and Stern, C. (1948) *Genetics*, 33, 263–272.

overcome by calculating the twinning rate in all delivered patients who booked before the 26th week of pregnancy since the diagnosis of twins and pregnancy complications due to twinning are rare before this time in pregnancy. Such an analysis was carried out in University College Hospital, Ibadan, where the twinning rate, even in booked patients, is very high (approximately 80/1000 maternities) and the results gave an incidence of twinning similar to that in a population in a rural area in Western Nigeria (Igbo-Ora) which is representative of the general population.

Another method (mentioned earlier) which may be used in deriving the twinning rate in a population relates to the proportion of twins which are monochorionic in that population. For example, the twinning rate in Western Nigeria (approx. 45/1000 maternities for Igbo-Ora) is approximately four times that in the U.K. (approx. 11/1000 maternities) and the proportion of twins with monochorionic placentae in Western Nigeria (approx. five per cent) is one-fourth that found in populations in the U.K. (approx. 20 per cent). Thus, it appears that there is an inverse relationship between twinning rates and monochorionic rates in populations. This relationship can be expressed thus:

$$\frac{\text{Twinning rate in a population } n_1}{\text{Twinning rate in a population } n_2} = \frac{\% \text{ of MCH in twins in } n_2}{\% \text{ of MCH in twins in } n_1}$$

It appears that this relationship, to which attention has already been drawn (Nylander, 1970d) may be used in estimating the twinning rate in a population if the proportion of twins with monochorionic placentae can be found. Thus, if the proportion of twins with monochorionic placentae in a population is, say, 10% the twinning rate in that population may be calculated thus, using the data for Western Nigeria given above:

$$\frac{\text{Twinning rate in } n_1}{45} = \frac{5}{10}$$

(approx.) Twinning in $n_1 = \dfrac{5 \times 45}{10} = 22.5/1000$ maternities

ETHNIC DIFFERENCES

Much has been written about the rates of twinning in different ethnic groups in many countries. For example, Eriksson and Fellman (1967) in their report, which called attention to the different twinning trends between the Swedes and Finns, mentioned certain Finnish tribes which have a much higher twinning incidence (16.3 per 1000 maternities) than the rest of the population. Similarly, differences have been reported in some other countries, e.g. France (Bulmer, 1960) and Israel (Modan et al, 1968).

In tropical Africa where there are usually *several* ethnic groups in a country, this variation of twinning incidence with ethnicity becomes even more important, since twinning rates may vary widely in different sections of the same population according to their ethnic groups. For example, in a recent study in a Western Nigerian population (Nylander, 1970d) it was found that

Table 5.4 *Comparison of the incidence of multiple births in some populations in Nigeria, the U.K. and U.S.A.; expected incidence, calculated by Hellin's formula is shown in parenthesis.*

	Total number of maternities	Incidence (per 1000 maternities)			Reference
		Twins	Triplets	Quadruplets	
Nigeria					
Igbo-Ora	6160	47.0	1.62 (2.2)	—	Present study
Ibadan					
Adeoyo and U.C.H.	21 940	66.5	1.78 (4.4)	0.06 (0.29)	Present study
Ilesha					
Wesley Guild Hospital	10 800	76.1	1.94 (5.8)	—	Mulligan (1970)
U.K.					
England and Wales	5956 220	11.4	0.10 (0.13)	0.0015 (0.0015)	Registrar General (1963–69)
U.S.A.					
White[a]	23 751 611	10.0	0.09 (0.10)	0.001 (0.001)	Statistical Bulletin of Metropolitan Life Insurance Co. (1960)
Negro[a]	3946 146	13.4	0.14 (0.18)	0.0018 (0.0024)	
Sweden	3188 149	13.6	0.13 (0.18)	0.0016 (0.0025)	Herrlin and Hauge (1967)

[a] Figures refer to multiple births where at least one infant survived.
Reprinted from Nylander (1971c) with kind permission of the editors of *Annals of Human Genetics* and Cambridge University Press.

the twinning rate in the major ethnic group (which constitutes 85 per cent of the population) was 45 per 1000 maternities. The twinning rates in the other ethnic groups varied between 20 and 45 per 1000 maternities.

ZYGOSITY

The recent study of twinning rate in Western Nigeria has confirmed the high dizygotic twinning rate (approx. 44/1000 maternities), the monozygotic twinning rate (approx. 4.1/1000 maternities in Igbo-Ora) being similar to that in the U.K. and U.S.A. (4.2/1000 maternities). This finding is in agreement with the results of other investigations in different parts of the world (Bulmer, 1960; Hytten and Leitch, 1964; Shipley et al, 1967, etc.) which indicates that the monozygotic twinning rate in all populations varies very little (between 3 to 4/1000 maternities) and that it is variation in dizygotic twinning rates which accounts for the different twinning rates in populations. This is well shown in Tables 5.1, 5.2 and 5.3. From these tables it will be seen that countries in Asia with extremely low twinning rates (relative to those in Africa) still have monozygotic twinning rates which are not very different from those in other populations. The monozygotic twinning rates which have been reported for many of the populations in Africa and India are higher than expected (Bulmer, 1960; Cox, 1963, etc.). This is most likely to be due to the fact that such twinning rates have been obtained from hospital populations; the data are therefore likely to be subject to varying degrees of hospital bias.

INCIDENCE OF TRIPLETS AND HIGHER MULTIPLE BIRTHS

If the twinning rate in a population is known the expected incidence of triplet and quadruplet births can be calculated by using Hellin's hypothesis (1895) which states that, if the frequency of twinning in a population is n the frequency of triplets will be n^2 and that of quadruplets will be n^3. Other authors who have confirmed these results are Zeleny (1921), Dahlberg (1926) and Greulich (1930). Hellin made no distinction between the different types of triplets and quadruplets and did not take into account the variation which occurred with maternal age. Some authors (Jenkins, 1927; Allen and Firschein, 1957; Bulmer, 1958; Allen, 1960) have proposed various modifications to this 'law' or other methods to rectify this omission and to correct the small discrepancies between observed and expected frequencies when multiple birth frequencies are calculated from national statistics of some countries by applying this law.

There are many reports from countries in Europe and the United States of the incidence of triplets and higher multiple births, most of which have been computed from national statistics. In developing countries, in the absence of national statistics, such reliable data are not usually available. In a recent study (Nylander, 1971c) of triplets and higher multiple births however, it was possible to estimate the frequency of triplets in Western Nigeria by comparing the rate in a total population in a rural area (Igbo-Ora) with those obtained from hospital populations in other parts of Western Nigeria (Nylander, 1971c). The triplet rate in the hospital populations was found to be generally higher than that for the total population presumably because of varying degrees of hospital bias (Table 5.4). The expected triplet and quadruplet rates in the Nigerian and other populations have also been calculated by applying Hellin's 'law' (Table 5.4). The observed rates are all lower than the expected rate, but the difference may not be significant because of the small sample size. If the abortion rate in triplet conceptions were higher than in twins, then this could result in the observed number of triplets being less than that expected from Hellin's law but there is no adequate evidence on this point.

It will be seen from Table 5.4 that the twinning rate in Igbo-Ora is approximately four times that in the populations in the U.K. and U.S.A. When triplet rates are compared, that in Igbo-Ora (1.6/1000 maternities) is approximately 16 (i.e., 4^2) times the rate in the U.K. and U.S.A. (0.19 to 0.1/1000 maternities). The multiple birth rates shown for Sweden are slightly higher than those in the populations in the U.K. and U.S.A. but the twinning rate in Igbo-Ora is approximately 3.5 times that in Sweden, and the triplet rate is approximately 12.5 (3.5^2) times. Similarly, a comparison between the multiple birth rates in Igbo-Ora and U.S.A. (Negro populations) shows that the Igbo-Ora twinning and triplet rates are approximately 3.5 and 12.5 (3.5^2) times the corresponding rates in the Negro populations in the U.S.A. A comparison between the multiple birth rates in the hospital populations in Western Nigeria and those of the other countries shown in Table 5.1, does not give similar results, presumably because of varying degrees in hospital bias in twin and triplet maternities in the Nigerian population. Owing to the small numbers of quadruplets in the Western Nigerian population, it is difficult to make similar comparisons for this order of multiple births in Western Nigeria and the other countries.

Thus, by comparing the multiple birth rates between Igbo-Ora and other countries in Table 5.1, a relationship can be demonstrated between twinning and triplet rates in two different populations which may be expressed in general terms as $\dfrac{m_1}{m_2} = \left(\dfrac{n_1}{n_2}\right)^2$ where m_1 and m_2 represent triplet rates in population 1 and population 2 respectively, and n_1 and n_2, twinning rates in these populations.

CHAPTER 6

Factors which Influence Twinning Rates

P. P. S. NYLANDER

MATERNAL AGE AND PARITY

The association between maternal age and parity and the incidence of twinning has been known for a long time. For example, Duncan (1865) found that twin pregnancy was more likely in older and more parous women. Other authors (Guttmacher, 1937; McArthur, 1949) reported similar findings but they were unable to decide whether age and parity were separate factors. More recent studies (Anderson, 1956; Bulmer, 1959b; Millis, 1959; Registrar General, England and Wales, 1958; Eriksson and Fellman, 1967) have shown that the twinning incidence increases with maternal age up to a peak at 35 to 39 years, and thereafter falls; and also that there is a continuous gradual rise of twinning incidence with birth order, independent of maternal age. The increase in twinning rates with maternal age and parity was found to be due to an increase in the dizygotic twinning rates, there being very little variation in the monozygotic rates. While there has been general agreement on the strong correlation of twinning rates (especially dizygotic twinning rates) with maternal age, a few authors have been unable to demonstrate any definite relation between twinning rates and the number of previous births (Dahlberg, 1926; Lamy et al, 1955; Gedda, 1961). Another study which shows some differences from the general findings in most studies in Caucasian populations is that of Myrianthopoulos (1970) who found that the incidence of twinning rose steeply with maternal age up to a peak at the age group 30 to 34 years after which it fell, but rose again after the age group 35 to 39.

A recent study of twinning in a Caucasian population (Aberdeen, Scotland) and an African population (Ibadan, Western Nigeria) has also shown that twinning rates vary with maternal age and parity. In the Aberdeen population the incidence of twinning rose with maternal age to a peak in the age group

98

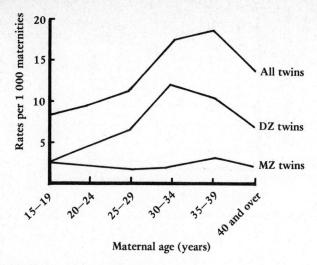

Figure 6.1. Influence of age on the incidence of twinning in Aberdeen.

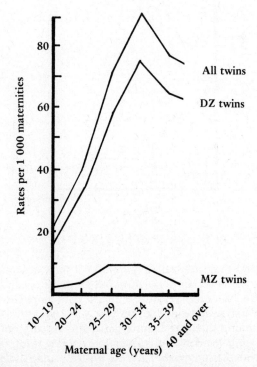

Figure 6.2. Influence of age on the incidence of twinning in Nigeria.

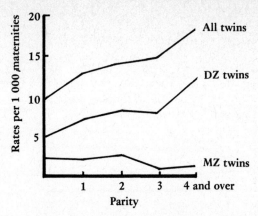

Figure 6.3. Influence of parity on the incidence of twinning in Aberdeen.

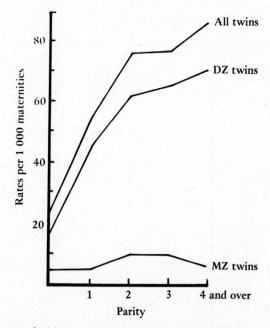

Figure 6.4. Influence of parity on the incidence of twinning in Nigeria.

35 to 39 years and thereafter fell (Figure 6.1). There was a similar rise with maternal age in the Nigerian population but the peak occurred in an earlier age group (30 to 34 years) (Figure 6.2). In both populations it was the variation in the dizygotic twinning rate that was largely responsible for the variation in twinning rate, the monozygotic rate varying only slightly with age. The increasing incidence of dizygotic twinning with maternal age is probably due to increasing ovarian activity possibly under hormonal stimulus causing increased double ovulation, the fall in incidence occurring because of

exhaustian of the Graafian follicles as the menopause approaches. Since women usually begin childbearing much earlier in Nigeria than in Europe, it is possible that ovarian activity reaches a peak at an earlier age in Nigeria, thus accounting for the difference in pattern between the Ibadan and Aberdeen populations. The twinning rates also increased with parity, in both populations (Figures 6.3 and 6.4). Again, it was variation in the dizygotic twinning rates that was responsible for the variation in the overall twinning rates. It was also found that the variation with parity was independent of that with age and vice versa, since the rise in twinning rate with parity was found to occur in each maternal age group and vice versa.

HEIGHT

The relation of twinning rates to height of the mother has been studied by some authors (Tchouriloff, 1877; McArthur, 1942; Anderson, 1956; Nylander, 1971a; Campbell, Campbell and MacGillivray, 1974). Anderson in a study of twinning in Aberdeen women during the years 1943 to 1952, showed that there was an increase in twinning incidence with height of the mother. Campbell et al, studying heights in the same population, confirmed these findings for women who delivered in Aberdeen during the period 1950 to 69, but not during the intermediate period 1960 to 64. They found that there was a greater number of tall women with twins compared to singleton pregnancies and this was seen particularly in primigravidae but also applied in multiparae. In the study by Nylander (1971a), the rise of twinning rate with height was found to be due to variation in the dizygotic twinning rate (Table 6.1).

Table 6.1. *Incidence of monozygotic and dizygotic twinning in relation to maternal height in Aberdeen (1950 to 1965).*

	No. of twin maternities	Twinning rates per 1000 maternities in maternal height groups		
		Short (under 5′1″)	Medium (5′1″–5′3¾″)	Tall (5′4″ and over)
MZ twins	95	1.9	1.8	2.2
DZ twins	345	6.5	6.9	7.3
Twins with undetermined zygosity	168	3.5	3.3	3.4
All twins	608	12.0	12.0	12.9

The investigation of twinning rates and maternal heights in an African population (Ibadan, Nigeria) showed that there was a marked gradient of twinning incidence with height, the taller women having the highest twinning rate. The gradient persisted after standardisation for maternal age and parity and was due to a variation in the dizygotic twinning rate, the monozygotic rate remaining fairly constant (Table 6.2). The height gradient which can be seen in this table in women with twins whose zygosity had not been determined is probably due to a high proportion of dizygotic twins in this group. The lower dizygotic twinning rate in the shorter women may be due to the

Table 6.2. *Incidence of twinning in relation to maternal height in Ibadan (1967 to 1968).*

	No. of twin maternities	Twinning rates per 1000 maternities in maternal height groups		
		Short (under 5′1″)	Medium (5′1″–5′3¾″)	Tall (5′4″ and over)
MZ twins	84	5.1	4.3	4.3
DZ twins	874	44.7	50.7	57.6
Twins with undetermined zygosity	56	1.6	2.7	5.4
All twins	1014	51.4	57.7	67.4

possibility that some women living in these conditions are not only stunted in growth but also under-nourished, a factor normally associated with a lowered twinning rate.

Since height is partly determined by nutrition, especially during early years of life, it would be expected that if twinning rates increased with maternal height a similar relation could be found between twinning rates and nutrition. There is evidence from studies in animals that a rise in the plane of nutrition is accompanied by a rise in the litter size (Wallace, 1951; Hammond, 1952). Furthermore, Bulmer (1959a) showed that there was a fall in the dizygotic twinning rate in some countries in Europe during the years of deprivation during the war, followed by a rise later when conditions returned to normal. Bulmer (1970) attributes the fall in dizygotic twinning rate, which occurs with undernutrition, to diminished secretion of gonadotrophin by the pituitary, known to occur in experimental animals following prolonged under-feeding (Burrows, 1949; Keys et al, 1950).

WEIGHT

The effects of nutrition are also reflected by the body weight so that the incidence of twinning might be expected to be higher in obese women if nutrition is a factor in twinning. Campbell and co-workers (1974) divided 158 primigravidae with twin pregnancies into thin, normal and fat groups according to the weight for height centile categories of Kemsley, Billewicz and Thomson (1962). In women having twins there were only 10 per cent thin compared with the expected 25 per cent while there was an excess of about seven per cent in the normal build and obese groups. There is therefore a greater tendency for twins to occur in women of normal or obese build than in thin women.

SOCIAL CLASS

In the few studies that have been conducted, the evidence for variation in twinning rates with social class appears to be conflicting. Daly (quoted by Anderson, 1956) analysing 1949 figures for England and Wales could not show any gradient in twinning rates with social class. This finding has recently been confirmed by Nylander (1971a) and by Campbell, Campbell and Mac-Gillivray (1974) in their study of twinning in the Aberdeen population. However, Smith (1966) analysing the figures for Scotland for the years 1962 to 1964 showed that there was an association of dizygotic twinning with social class in each maternal age group, the less favoured social class experiencing the highest incidence. He was not able to show a social class gradient within each parity group and suggests that the association may be due to a higher fertility rate in the lower social classes, assuming that the incidence of twinning is higher in more fertile women. The probable reason for the higher incidence in lower social class women is that they are of higher parity.

In the investigation of social class in the Nigerian population, the patients who delivered in two major hospitals in Ibadan have been divided primarily into two broad groups—those who are literate and those who are not. The literate group has been further subdivided into two groups A and B. Group A includes wives of professionals, senior university staff, teachers, typists and white collar workers, and group B consists mainly of manual workers. The illiterate group constituting about 60 per cent of the population is comprised mainly of peasants and traders belonging to the lowest social class C. Table 6.3 shows that the rates of twinning in groups A and B were 28 and 30 per 1000 maternities respectively compared with 62 per 1000 maternities in the lowest social class. The dizygotic twinning rate showed a gradient between the three groups from 19/1000 maternities in group A to 54/1000 maternities in group C, but the monozygotic twinning rates for the three groups (6, 2 and 4 per 1000 maternities respectively) showed no such gradient.

Table 6.3. *Incidence of twinning by social class: Ibadan.*

	Social class		
	A	B	C
Incidence per 1000 maternities	28	30	62
No. of maternities	1991	1150	4320

This finding of a much higher twinning rate in the illiterate women than in the literate women appears to be inconsistent with the findings in relation to maternal height viz. that the women who are short in stature (and are more likely to be of a lower social class) have a lower twinning rate than tall women (Tables 6.1 and 6.2). A further analysis has therefore been done to investigate the relation of twinning rates with social class and heights. In this analysis, data for mothers from the largest ethnic group (the Yorubas) who

Table 6.4. *Incidence of twinning by social class and height in Yoruba women delivered in University College Hospital and Oke-Offa Hospital.*

	Literate group			Illiterate group		
	Short	Medium	Tall	Short	Medium	Tall
Incidence per 1000 maternities	31	26	30	58	74	65
No. of maternities	541	1200	631	1125	1639	675

delivered in the two hospitals have been used. The results are shown in Table 6.4. Again the twinning rates are higher in the illiterate group of women than in the literate group. There is no gradient in twinning rates between short, medium or tall women in the literate group of women, the rates being 31, 26 and 30 per 1000 maternities respectively, but in the illiterate mothers the twinning rates for the medium and tall women (74 and 65 per 1000 maternities respectively) are higher than that for the short women, which is 58/1000 maternities.

The finding that there is no gradient of twinning with height in women in the upper social classes (the literate women) is probably because the shorter women in this group are smaller as a result of hereditary factors and not because of undernutrition. It appears that it is in the illiterate women (most of whom are stunted in growth, probably because of malnutrition) that the gradient of twinning and height occurs (the medium and tall women having a higher twinning rate than the shorter women). Again, it is the variation in the dizygotic twinning rate that is responsible for the gradient in twinning rates and social class in Ibadan; there is no such gradient in the monozygotic twinning rate.

SEASONAL VARIATION

Some twinning studies have suggested that the incidence of twinning varies at different times of the year. Timonen and Carpen (1968) found a more marked seasonal variation in multiple than in singleton pregnancy conceptions in Finland and have suggested that this was related to the ratio between daylight and darkness at different times of the year. The alteration in this ratio was thought to induce over-stimulation of the hypothalamic-hypophyseal system. However, their data included only liveborn deliveries and the exclusion of stillbirths might have created a bias. Smith (1966) in his analysis of data for Scotland did not find any seasonal variation in the incidence of twinning. The findings in the Aberdeen study indicated that there was a rise in the incidence of twin births during Spring (Nylander, 1975, unpublished data) but the increase was not significant.

Knox and Morley (1960) and Cox (1963) studying twin births in Imesi, Western Nigeria and in Eastern Nigeria have suggested that there is a correlation between the twinning incidence and the rainfall and temperature in Western Nigeria. The data however were collected from hospital patients and the authors did not investigate the possibility that the utilisation of hospital facilities might vary at different times of the year. For example, mothers expecting twins and therefore more likely to have complications of pregnancy or labour, will endeavour to enter hospital whatever the weather or difficulties of transport, whereas other mothers may be more easily deterred from going into hospital in the rainy season.

In a recent study of seasonal variation of twinning in Western Nigeria (Nylander, 1975, unpublished data) the twinning rate in the Ibadan hospitals during the rainy season (May to October) was found to be higher than that during the dry season (November to April). This finding is in agreement with that of Knox and Morley (1960) and Cox (1963). However, when the data for Igbo-Ora (which represents a total population with no bias such as is seen in hospital populations) were analysed it was found that the incidence of twinning was higher during the dry season, although the difference was not significant. The findings in the Ibadan hospitals and in Knox and Morley (1960) and Cox's (1963) investigations are very likely due to the difference in utilisation of hospital services by twin mothers and singleton mothers during the rainy and dry seasons.

BLOOD GROUPS

There is no conclusive evidence of a direct association between blood groups and the incidence of twinning. The finding of a high twinning rate in areas of high B blood group frequency in France (Vallois, 1949; Bulmer, 1960) is probably a reflection of ethnic differences due to migration. Other authors who have supported the hypothesis of an association of twinning incidence with blood groups are Gedda (1961), Osborne and De George (1957), and Bolognesi and Milani-Comparetti (1970). The last two authors postulate that mothers who belong to group O have a higher incidence of twinning. In both the Aberdeen and Ibadan studies, no significant association of twinning with blood groups was found.

FERTILITY AND FECUNDABILITY

It is believed by some that there is a relation between twinning and fecundability (i.e., the ease with which a woman conceives). Bulmer (1959b) found that there is a higher twinning rate among women who conceived during the first three months of marriage than among women who did not conceive until later. Allen and Schachter (1971) have suggested that a possible explanation for this finding is that women who conceive most easily are also prone to bear twins. These authors have also suggested that the twinning peak which occurred in the United States in 1946 may be explained by the assumption that dizygotic twins were conceived more promptly than singletons following the return of fathers from military service, thus indicating that prompt conception and twin proneness might be associated. It is possible, however, to explain these two findings (a high twinning rate in the first few months of marriage and in the first few months after the return of father from military service, in the U.S.A.) by assuming that more frequent sexual intercourse is likely to occur during these 'first few months'. It is possible that at double ovulation only one of the ova may sometimes be fertilised; more frequent intercourse is likely to result in the fertilisation of the other ovum. However, Eriksson and Fellman's (1967) findings of a higher twinning rate in illegitimate maternities in Finland lends some support to the theory that high fecundity and twin proneness may be associated, since, as suggested by Allen and Schachter (1971), it is likely that it is the highly fecundable women who get 'caught' by pregnancy. In the Aberdeen study it was also found that there was a higher twinning rate in illegitimate maternities (14.9 per 1000 maternities) compared to the rate in the general population. Furthermore, in every maternal age and parity group the twinning rates were higher for illegitimate maternities than the legitimate maternities.

SECULAR TRENDS IN TWINNING INCIDENCE

Many investigations have drawn attention to the changes which have occurred in twinning rates in different countries over the past decades. MacGillivray (1970) has shown that the twinning incidence in Scotland has declined steadily since 1958. The incidence for England and Wales has also declined since 1958 (James, 1972). Similar trends have been found in many other countries: Italy, Holland, Norway, Sweden, Denmark, Switzerland, Belgium, New Zealand, Australia, Portugal, Spain and Japan (James, 1972). In the United States, there was an earlier decline in the twinning incidence from 1933 to 1950 (Jeanneret and MacMahon, 1962) after which the incidence has remained fairly static. In Finland, however, the incidence of twinning has risen steadily since the beginning of the present century (Eriksson and Fellman, 1967).

In all these countries, it was the dizygotic twinning rates that had changed, the monozygotic rate remaining fairly constant. The cause of the changing dizygotic incidence has been attributed to various factors: changing maternal age and parity distribution, a decrease in the proportion of highly fertile women because of the widespread use of contraceptives (Parkes, 1969; Allen and Schachter, 1971), improved socioeconomic conditions, earlier sexual maturation (which is believed by some to be associated with an increase in twinning rate (Škerlj, 1939), the use of hormonal and pesticide substances in agriculture (James, 1972). These factors, however, cannot entirely account for the changing incidence, and in many cases the cause still remains obscure. The possibility of environmental factors influencing twinning rates through alterations in the output of pituitary hormones has been discussed in Chapter 4, together with the results of an investigation into the relationship between serum gonadotrophin levels and twinning.

In the absence of national vital statistics it is difficult to know what secular trends have occurred in twinning rates in populations in tropical Africa. The recent study in Igbo-Ora (Western Nigeria), however, suggests that the twinning incidence has been rising over the last few years probably as a result of the improved health facilities and improved nutrition in the area over the last decade.

CHAPTER 7

Physiological Changes in Twin Pregnancy

I. MACGILLIVRAY

The physiological changes which occur in singleton pregnancy are so dramatic that they would be considered pathological in the non-pregnant female. This is amply demonstrated by reference to the values reported in *Diagnostic Indices in Pregnancy* (1973). It is therefore necessary to be aware of these changes so that misinterpretations of physical and biochemical findings do not occur. But even in this excellent reference book no mention is made of the even more dramatic changes which occur in multiple pregnancies and it is all the more essential that the changes should be recognised as being within the normal physiological range. However, as complications are so very common in twin pregnancies, particularly if they continue near to term, it is possible that multiple pregnancies should not be considered physiological in the human. Indeed, as long ago as 1887 Matthews Duncan wrote "the rarity of a plural birth in woman and the increased danger to both mother and offspring in these circumstances render such an event in a certain limited sense a disease or an abnormality".

All of the organs and systems of the body are affected by pregnancy. Some of the changes occur very early in pregnancy while others develop gradually during the pregnancy. The range of physiological normality in multiple pregnancy is somewhat difficult to determine because complications are so common, the diagnosis of twin pregnancy is often not made until late in pregnancy and also because a truly normal pregnancy in terms of absence of complications and the production of two good sized babies is indeed rare as some degree of intrauterine growth retardation occurs in most multiple pregnancies.

However, the changes which occur in pregnancies that are not complicated by any obvious obstetrical or medical condition are now being studied in greater detail and several parameters of physiological change have been recorded. In some animals it is normal to have more than one in the litter and the combined weight of the litter-mates is related to the maternal size. In view of the relative rarity of multiple pregnancies in humans it is usual to consider these multiple pregnancies as abnormal, but it seems unjustifiable to consider multiple pregnancy in the human as an atavistic reversion. In some animals, such as the sheep, twinning is more likely to occur if there has been increased nutrition. It is doubtful if this is true of the human as there is no evidence to suggest that women having twin pregnancies have a better diet than women having singleton pregnancies, but it has been observed recently (Campbell, Campbell and MacGillivray, 1974) that women who have twin pregnancies have a higher pre-pregnant weight for height than those having a singleton pregnancy.

As in singleton pregnancies it seems probable that in twin pregnancies all systems are affected and the degree to which they are affected is probably greater than in singleton pregnancies.

CHANGES IN THE BLOOD AND CARDIOVASCULAR SYSTEM

It has been clearly established by many workers that in singleton pregnancies there is an increase in total blood volume but that the plasma volume increase is relatively greater than the increase in the red cell mass so that there is a lower haematocrit and haemoglobin concentration in normal pregnancy than in the non-pregnant. The changes which occur in twin pregnancy compared to singleton pregnancy are even more dramatic. Rovinsky and Jaffin (1965) found a mean value of four litres of plasma volume in singleton pregnancies between 37 and 40 weeks gestation compared to a mean of 4.7 litres at the same duration of pregnancy in seven twin pregnancies. The value in single pregnancies showed a rise of 48 per cent above the normal non-pregnant values near term and in the twin pregnancies the values rose to a peak of 67 per cent above the normal non-pregnant levels. However, these authors did not differentiate their subjects into primigravidae and multi-gravidae. A study of primigravidae (MacGillivray, Campbell and Duffus, 1971) with twin pregnancies confirmed the finding that there was a greater increase in plasma volume in the twin pregnancies than in the singleton. At 34 weeks gestation in the singletons the plasma volume was 3.8 litres compared to 4.3 litres in the twin pregnancies. The differentiation of parity is important because plasma volume in singletons was found to be 4.2 litres in women in their second pregnancies compared to 3.7 litres in their first pregnancies at the same duration of pregnancy (Campbell and MacGillivray, 1972). There was significant correlation between the serum volumes and baby weight in both pregnancies. However, in twin pregnancies, although there is a slightly greater increase in plasma volume in the multiparous women compared to primigravid women with twin pregnancies, there was no correlation between serum volume and birthweight in the primigravid women, although there was in the multiparous women (Campbell, Campbell and Mac-Gillivray, 1975). It is difficult to understand why there is a correlation between baby weight and serum volume in singleton primigravidae and multigravidae, in multigravid twin pregnancies but not in primigravid twin pregnancies. It might be that in spite of the marked increase in the plasma volume the uterus and uterine blood flow cannot expand sufficiently to allow the growth of large enough babies to correspond with the serum volume.

In their series MacGillivray, Campbell and Duffus (1971) found a mean total red cell volume of 2063 ml in twin pregnancy compared to 1694 ml in singleton pregnancy at 34 weeks. This compares favourably with Rovinsky and Jaffin (1966a) who found a red cell volume of 1799 ml between 33 and 36 weeks in singletons and 2056 ml in twin pregnancies. Although there is this marked increase in red cell volume it is relatively not as great as the increase in the plasma volume so that the haemodilution which is seen in singleton pregnancies is even more marked in multiple pregnancies.

The increase in serum volume also has the effect of reducing the total protein concentration (see Table 7.1) but there was no alteration in the total circulating intravascular protein mass in twin pregnancy compared to singletons (MacGillivray, Campbell and Duffus, 1971). There is no significant change in serum sodium, potassium or chloride levels and the serum osmolality does not differ from singleton pregnancy (see Table 7.1).

Table 7.1. *Some serum values at 38 weeks gestation.*

	Singleton pregnancies	*Twin pregnancies*
Protein concentration (g/100 ml)	6.1	5.5
Intravascular protein mass (g)	232.9	238.0
Serum sodium (mEq/l)	141.8	137.1
Serum potassium (mEq/l)	4.0	3.9
Serum chloride (mEq/l)	110.0	110.3
Serum osmolality (mosmoles/kg)	280[a]	285.0

[a] Quoted from Robertson (1969).

The coagulation changes have been studied in a small series of twin pregnancies by Condie (1974). No pattern of difference from normal singleton pregnancy was found in plasminogen, fibrin-fibrinogen degradation products, anti-thrombin (III), alpha I anti-trypsin or alpha II macroglobulin but the plasma fibrinogen levels whether measured by the thrombin clot method or by the heat precipitation method from 24 weeks gestation onwards remained significantly higher than the curve for normal singleton pregnancies.

Using Evans blue dye in the indicator dilution technique Rovinsky and Jaffin (1966a) found that in singleton pregnancies the mean cardiac output rose from 5.87 litres per minute in non-pregnant controls to 8.58 litres per minute between 25 and 28 weeks gestation and then fell progressively to normal levels at term. In twin pregnancy the cardiac output rose to 9.01 between 21 and 24 weeks and fell progressively to 6.93 between 37 and 40 weeks. As the measurements were probably made with the patients lying supine it is likely that the fall in cardiac output estimated towards the end of pregnancy is fallacious. However, it does seem that in twin pregnancy there is a greater cardiac output than in singleton pregnancy. They also found that the increase in the cardiac rate of 15 per cent, the mean cardiac stroke volume of 30 per cent and the mean circulation time of 18 per cent were of the same order in both single and twin pregnancies.

The blood pressure in singleton pregnancies falls below non-pregnant levels early in pregnancy and remains at this level until the last trimester when it rises again (MacGillivray, Rose and Rowe, 1969). Twenty per cent of primigravidae have a rise in blood pressure in the third trimester to 90 mm or more and this is associated with proteinuria in about five per cent of cases. In twin pregnancies, on the other hand, in late pregnancy there is a rise to 90 mm or more in 50 per cent and this is associated with proteinuria in about 20 per cent. The levels of blood pressure in mid-pregnancy have been compared in singleton and twins by Campbell, Campbell and MacGillivray (1975) and there appears to be a lower level of diastolic blood pressure in twin pregnancies at this stage than in singleton pregnancies. It is not clear, however, whether the rise in blood pressure towards the end of pregnancy is pathological and probably in many cases it is not.

The blood flow to the uterus, kidneys and skin is increased in singleton pregnancy and although the changes have not been measured it is probable that they are increased even more in multiple pregnancies.

There have been few studies of blood and cardiovascular changes in more multiple pregnancies than twins, but in a study of a quadruplet pregnancy (Fullerton et al, 1965) there was a very considerable increase in plasma volume up to 5990 ml at 34 weeks and the red cell volume increased to 2795 ml.

RESPIRATORY FUNCTION IN TWIN PREGNANCY

During pregnancy there is a considerable increase in the volume of air breathed each minute due to the increase in tidal volume with little or no increase in respiratory rate. The vital capacity of the lungs is probably unchanged by pregnancy but the residual volume is reduced about 20 per cent, the functional residual capacity is reduced 18 per cent and the total lung volume is slightly reduced. In a small series of twin pregnancies Templeton and Kelman (1974) have found that there is an even greater increase in the tidal volume.

RENAL FUNCTION

In normal singleton pregnancies there is a dilation of the ureter above the level of the pelvic brim. This occurs in the early weeks of pregnancy but is no longer considered to be due to the action of progesterone as ureteric tone and contractile pressure have been shown to be normal or above normal in pregnancy. The effect is now presumed to be due to pressure. The kidneys enlarge slightly during pregnancy and there is an increase in the renal blood flow from about 500 ml per minute to 700 ml per minute. The glomerular filtration rate is considerably increased during pregnancy from about 90 ml per minute to 150 ml per minute. The filtration fraction, i.e. the proportion of plasma filtered, is also raised since the glomerular filtration rate rises proportionally more than renal plasma flow. Urea, creatinine, uric acid, amino acids and vitamins such as folic acid are excreted in greater amounts than in the non-pregnant woman. It is not known whether there is a greater excretion of the substances in twin pregnancies, but presumably this is so because Swapp (1975) has demonstrated an increased glomerular filtration rate in twin pregnancy compared to singleton.

ALIMENTARY SYSTEM

There is considerable change in the alimentary system in terms of oesophageal reflux, hypochlorhydria, reduced gastric mobility and constipation in singleton pregnancies and these changes are probably aggravated in multiple pregnancies.

In singleton pregnancy the rate of return of bromsulphthalein from the liver to the plasma is increased and the rate of excretion of the dye from the liver cells is reduced compared with the non-pregnant state. The proportion of dye eliminated from the liver cells per minute into the bile is consequently reduced (Beazley and Tindall, 1966). In uncomplicated multiple pregnancies the bromsulphthalein test showed that changes occur in hepatic function similar to but greater than in singleton pregnancies. Fotheringham (1974) using a modification of the usual bromsulphthalein excretion test which yields more information than the standard test (Barber-Riley et al, 1961) found an increased transfer from plasma to liver in twins and she thought this was due to the greater plasma volume and cardiac output in twin pregnancies leading to an increased amount of blood passing through the liver per minute. She, like Tindall and Beazley (1966) however, found an increased transfer of dye from liver to plasma in twin pregnancies and thought this could be accounted for by an excess of binding of proteins by oestrogens or progesterone leading to an even greater return of unbound BSP in the plasma than in singleton pregnancies.

ENDOCRINE CHANGES

There have been few studies of endocrine changes in twin pregnancies and it can only be assumed that the changes occurring in singleton pregnancies such as the increase in cortisol, aldosterone and the increase in the total concentration of circulating thyroid hormone are even more marked in multiple pregnancies. The placental hormones oestrogen, progesterone and placental lactogen, as would be anticipated, are increased in twin pregnancies. The excretion of oestriol in the urine (Table 7.2) for example, is increased by about 50 per cent over the singleton values (MacGillivray and Campbell,

1975). Plasma oestriol values in twin pregnancy are similarly increased (Table 7.3) (Masson, 1974).

Table 7.2. *Mean urinary oestriol (mg/24 hours).*

	Weeks		
	30	*34*	*38*
Primigravidae			
Twins	16.17 ± 5.12 (15)	21.72 ± 10.49 (15)	27.67 ± 7.07 (6)
Singletons	10.8 ± 4.06 (38)	13.8 ± 4.45 (45)	19.4 ± 7.85 (44)
Multiparae			
Twins	20.91 ± 7.85 (29)	24.1 ± 8.14 (32)	33.54 ± 12.92 (13)
Singletons	10.2 ± 2.83 (18)	13.84 ± 3.81 (18)	23.33 ± 8.61 (18)

Table 7.3. *Mean plasma oestriol in twin pregnancies compared to singleton pregnancies.*

Weeks	*Twins*	*Singletons*
30	12 ± 3.4	9.19 ± 3.76
34	16.5 ± 3.3	13.02 ± 3.57
38	31.3 ± 3.0	15.5 ± 4.96

ENZYMES

Several enzymes show a progressively increasing concentration in pregnancy and measurements have been used as an indication of placental function, for example, heat-stable alkaline phosphatase and diamineoxidase. An appreciably higher level of serum diamine oxidase was found in twin pregnancies compared with normal singleton pregnancies by Ward, Whyley and Miller (1972).

WEIGHT GAIN

The weight gain in singleton pregnancies varies widely and it has been shown that there is a relationship between baby weight and the amount of weight gain in primigravidas. It would be expected that the weight gain in twin pregnancies would be greater than in singleton pregnancies and this was found by Campbell, Campbell and MacGillivray (1974), but surprisingly the weight gain in the first trimester was markedly greater than in the singletons (Table 7.4). As with singletons there was a relationship between the weight gain and weights of the twin babies. As well as an association between weight gain and baby weight a correlation has been found between total body water

Table 7.4. *Mean weekly weight gain (kg) in twin pregnancies in primigravidae compared to singleton pregnancies.*

Weeks	Twins	Singletons
13–20	0.60	0.42
20–30	0.54	0.47
30–36	0.64	0.40

and baby weight but only in primigravidae and not in parous women (Campbell and MacGillivray, 1975) (Figure 7.1). This is also true of twin pregnancies (Figure 7.2). There is a greater increase in total body water in twin pregnancies than in singletons and in primigravidae than in multi-

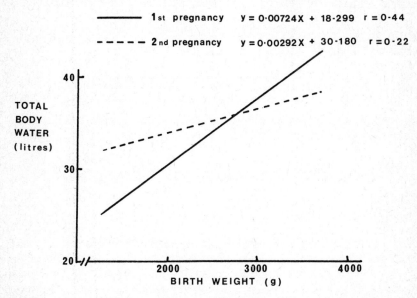

Figure 7.1. Total body water and baby weight in primigravid and parous singleton pregnancies.

parae (Figure 7.3). Thus the primigravida near term with a twin pregnancy has about 10 litres more water than the multipara with a singleton pregnancy. It is not surprising that the woman with a twin pregnancy has more water retention than one with a singleton pregnancy but it is not clear why the primigravida has more than the parous woman.

METABOLISM

Little is known about the increase in metabolism in twin pregnancies or about the nutrient requirements. About 2400 calories and 60 grams of protein are the amounts usually recommended for singleton pregnancy but it is not

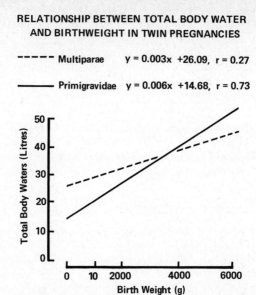

**RELATIONSHIP BETWEEN TOTAL BODY WATER
AND BIRTHWEIGHT IN TWIN PREGNANCIES**

- - - - - Multiparae $y = 0.003x + 26.09$, $r = 0.27$

———— Primigravidae $y = 0.006x + 14.68$, $r = 0.73$

Figure 7.2. Total body water and baby weight in primigravid and parous twin pregnancies.

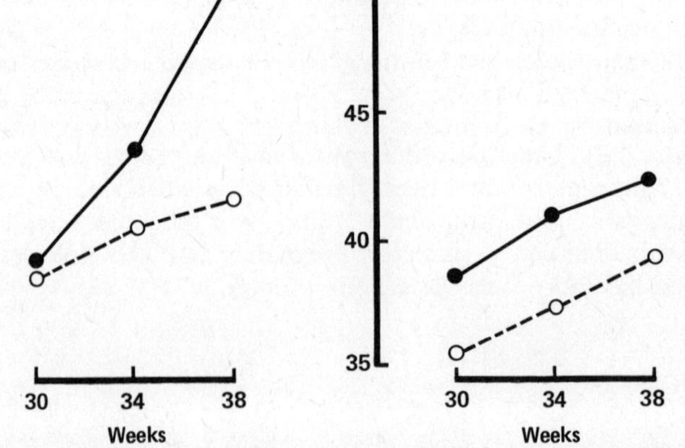

TOTAL BODY WATER IN TWIN AND SINGLETON PREGNANCIES

———— Twins   - - - - - Singletons

PRIMIGRAVIDAE   MULTIPARAE

Figure 7.3. Increase in total body water in singleton and twin and primigravid and parous pregnancies.

known how much this should be increased, if at all, for twin pregnancy. It is also not known whether supplements of calcium, folate, iron and vitamins are necessary. Disturbances of carbohydrate metabolism are common during pregnancy and this is particularly so in twin pregnancies. It is interesting to note that chemical gestational diabetes is more common in women having a twin pregnancy. All women with twin pregnancies should have a glucose tolerance test, preferably an intravenous one, performed in the last trimester of pregnancy.

INTRAUTERINE GROWTH OF THE BABIES

Curves of the intrauterine growth of monochorionic and dichorionic twins show that the weights of twins were progressively lower than median weights for single born infants during late gestation. Monochorionic twins were both smaller and had a greater intra-pair variation in birthweight than dichorionic pairs (Naeye et al, 1966). The findings confirmed those of McKeown and Record (1952) that fetal growth is independent of litter size until about the 30th week of gestation after which multiple fetuses show an increasing weight deficit. The median body weights of twins at the various gestational ages were similar to those observed by Guttmacher and Kohl (1958) but about 10 per cent less than those recorded by McKeown and Record. While most twins have a subnormal rate of growth during late gestation they have an accelerated rate of growth after birth reaching median levels for single born infants by 12 months of age (Naeye, 1964). This growth pattern supports McKeown's view that environmental rather than genetic factors are primarily responsible for the abnormal growth of twins in late fetal life. Kloosterman (1963) has pointed to the unequal exchange of plasma proteins as the most important factor in intra-pair variation of monozygous twins at birth. Naeye et al (1966) found that monochorionic twins were both smaller and had a greater intra-pair variation in birthweight than dichorionic pairs. Macmillan et al have recently found (1973) that twins with a relatively lower concentration of human placental lactogen in their placentas were of lower birthweight and birth length than their co-twins who had a relatively higher placental concentration of placental lactogen and they suggest that placental lactogen or chorionic somatomammotrophin production may represent an influence independent of general placental function in determining the weights of the babies.

CHAPTER 8

Diagnosis of Twin Pregnancy

I. MACGILLIVRAY

Although it is now recommended in some centres that a sonar scan should be performed early in pregnancy in all antenatal cases so that conditions such as multiple pregnancy can be diagnosed, it is likely that most twin pregnancies will continue to be diagnosed later in pregnancy, either because ultrasonic scanning is not available, or the clinician does not feel that this is a good routine, or again because some early multiple pregnancies might be missed on sonar scanning. It is for this last reason that it is important that clinicians in all centres should be aware of and alert to the signs suggestive of a multiple pregnancy. The greater size of multiple pregnancy compared to a singleton pregnancy is the feature which is most likely to draw the clinician's attention to the condition. Indeed, some women may draw the clinician's attention to the fact that they feel larger than they did in a previous singleton pregnancy.

The rate of increase in the height of the uterine fundus varies within fairly wide limits and there appears to be a variable increase in the individual patient with apparent spurts of growth at various times. It is difficult to be precise about when a difference in size can be noticed between a multiple and a singleton pregnancy, but the difference is not likely to be detected clinically much before 12 weeks. The fundal height is usually measured either in finger breadths or centimetres above the symphysis or below the xiphisternum or in relation to the umbilicus. The only reliable point from which measurements can be made is the symphysis pubis as the umbilicus is not a fixed point and the level of the fundus in relation to the xiphisternum is dependent on the height of the woman as well as on the duration of the pregnancy. Although it is dependent on the thickness of the abdominal wall and the lateral spread of the uterus the height of the fundus measured from the symphysis pubis preferably by means of a caliper or tape-measure gives quite a good approxi-

116

mation of the gestation length up to about 34 weeks of pregnancy. Thereafter the uterine size is not a good guide to length of gestation because it is more related to the size of the baby than gestation length. The height of the fundus at various gestation lengths is shown for a singleton and a multiple pregnancy for comparison in Figure 8.1.

The circumference of the abdomen can also be of some value in suspecting a twin pregnancy. This is possibly more useful after the 34th week of pregnancy. The circumference increases by about one inch for each week of gestation from 34 weeks up to 40 weeks when the circumference in a singleton pregnancy measures 40 inches at the level of the umbilicus.

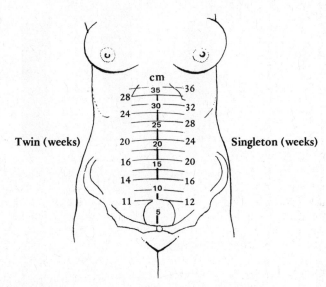

Figure 8.1. The height in cms of the fundus at various gestation lengths in weeks of singleton and twin pregnancies.

The amount of weight gain can also be a useful indicator of a multiple pregnancy, but again marked variations occur. In singletons the average weight gain is about a half pound a week up to 20 weeks and one pound a week thereafter until 36 weeks when the weight tends to level off. In a twin pregnancy, however, the weight gain is more marked in the first half of pregnancy and the increase in weight continues to be greater in the second half than in singleton pregnancies. The mean weekly weight gain in primigravid twin pregnancies is about the same between 13 and 20 weeks (598 g) as it is between 20 and 30 weeks (547 g) or 30 to 36 weeks (634 g) (Campbell, Campbell and MacGillivray, 1974). The graph of the weight gain for singleton and twin pregnancies illustrates these differences (Figure 8.2).

Apart from the increased size of the uterus the other feature which usually alerts the clinician to the condition is the presence of multiple fetal parts. There may be a suspiciously large number of small parts palpable, but this, of course, may be confused with the limbs in an occipito-posterior position. It is unusual to be able to palpate all four poles of the two fetuses but usually three can be made out. A twin pregnancy may be suspected if a head is clearly felt which seems to be small in relation to the amount of baby present. This is much more likely to be a twin pregnancy than a microcephalic fetus. Suspicions may be aroused if there is a fetal head in the pelvis and the

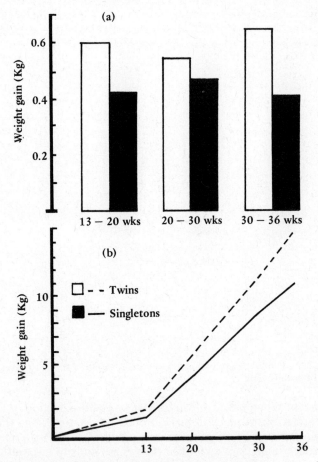

Figure 8.2. Maternal weight gain in singleton and twin pregnancies.

distance to the fundus seems too great for one baby length. Only three poles may be found because one head or breech may be deep in the pelvis. The fetal parts will be difficult to feel if there is an excess of liquor, but this in itself should arouse suspicions of the possibility of a multiple pregnancy.

The patient herself may have drawn attention to her condition because of some symptom such as discomfort under the costal margin due to pressure of the head of one of the babies, or because of oedema, dyspnoea, difficulty in walking, or excessive movements interfering with sleep.

Apart from mistakes in the estimation of the length of gestation, tumours in the pelvis, particularly ovarian cysts or fibromyomata and hydramnios are the most likely conditions to cause confusion in diagnosis. If a multiple pregnancy has not been suspected before delivery of the first baby, the differential diagnosis between a second twin and a fibromyoma or an ovarian cyst may only be made on exploration of the uterus.

Once the suspicion of multiple pregnancy has been aroused some assistance in diagnosis may be obtained from auscultation, but it is not a reliable method. The two fetal hearts must be auscultated simultaneously by two different observers and there must be a difference of 10 beats per minute between the two fetal hearts and even then the average of many counts should be taken before the diagnosis is made. It is usually considered useless for one observer to try to diagnose a twin pregnancy by auscultation.

Because it employs the detection of movement by the Doppler effect and is not dependent on sound the doptone is much more reliable in the diagnosis of a twin pregnancy than is the fetal stethoscope. When the fetal heart is detected on the doptone and the rate counted and then the direction of the doptone is changed and another fetal heart is recorded this can be accepted as evidence of a twin pregnancy. Even so it is preferable that two doptones are used simultaneously and it can be observed that the direction of the probes are different.

Fetal electrocardiography has been suggested by Hon and Hess (1960). However, others (Bernstine and Borkowski, 1955; Blondheim, 1947; Southern, 1954) have suggested that fetal electrocardiography may be of little use in the early detection of twin pregnancies. Electroencephalography was used by Novotny, Hass and Callagan (1959) to diagnose 21 twin pregnancies successfully between the 20th and 27th weeks of gestation. The reports on the use of ultrasound in the detection of twin pregnancies deal mainly with cases that were referred because of a suspicion of multiple pregnancy and the accuracy in diagnosis might decrease when a general population of pregnant women was screened (Figure 8.3). The problems of diagnosing multiple pregnancies by ultrasound have been dealt with by Donald (1974). He emphasises the limitations of two-dimensional visualisation and the difficulties of getting two, or particularly more, heads in the same sectional plane. Also the thorax may be confused with a head but this difficulty can be overcome by looking for the pulsations of the heart in the thorax. Twin pregnancies have been detected by ultrasound in the very early weeks of pregnancy, but the risk of false negative results in early pregnancy is very high (Figure 8.2). A very considerable feat was achieved by Campbell and Dewhurst (1970) in diagnosing quintuplets by ultrasound at the ninth week of pregnancy. It is usually recommended that screening for multiple pregnancies by ultrasound is best carried out at around 16 to 20 weeks. One of the strong arguments for routine ultrasonic scanning of all pregnant women is the detection of twin pregnancies and this should be possible in all pregnancies by the beginning of the third trimester.

Radiography readily reveals the presence of multiple fetuses from about 20 weeks onwards (Figure 8.4). Sonar scanning will also reveal the presence of multiple fetuses, but because of their mobility, it might not be possible to

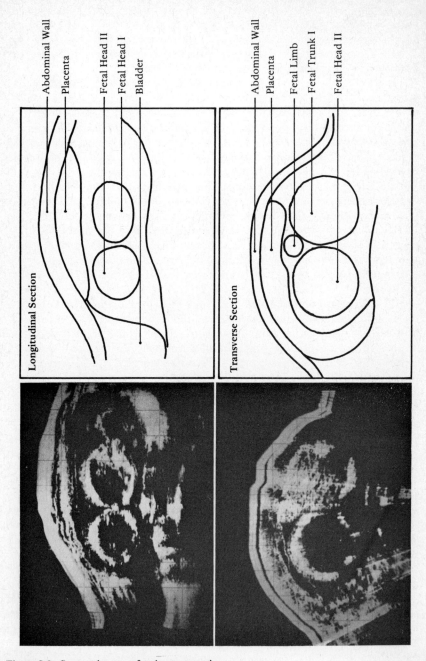

Figure 8.3. Sonar pictures of twin pregnancies.

diagnose with certainty the presence of many fetuses in utero. It is probably safer in cases of quadruplets or more to take an x-ray as this will not only show up the number of fetuses, but will also show any bony abnormalities which might be present (Figure 8.5).

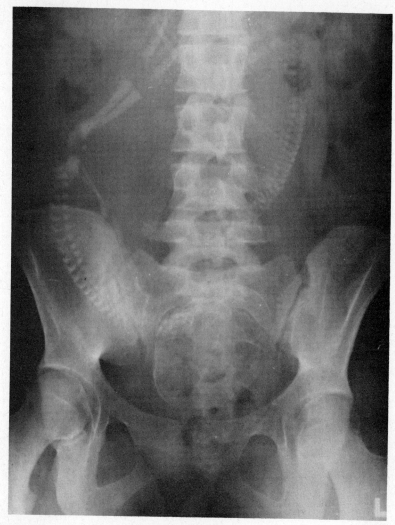

Figure 8.4. X-ray of twins with one anencephalic.

IMPORTANCE OF EARLY DIAGNOSIS

According to Law (1967) twins diagnosed during pregnancy tend to be heavier than twins not diagnosed before delivery. Twins who are not diagnosed during pregnancy are also of shorter gestation (Spurway, 1962). As twin

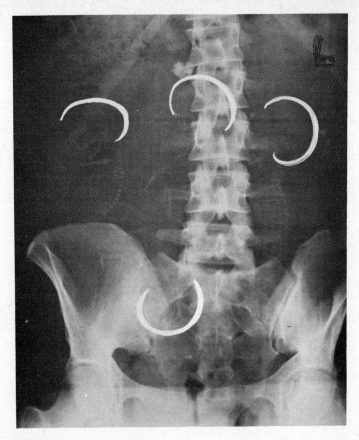

Figure 8.5. X-ray showing quadruplets.

babies tend to be growth-retarded it is obviously important that they should be of as great a gestational age as possible. If they are not diagnosed before the delivery there is the grave risk that ergometrine will be given with the delivery of the first baby and the second baby's oxygen supply will be reduced because of the shut-down of the placental blood flow due to the excessive uterine contraction. Delivery will also be made more difficult because of the closure of the cervix. If the twin pregnancy is not suspected the babies may be delivered in a situation where the intensive care for such small growth-retarded babies is not readily available. The earlier the twin pregnancy is diagnosed the greater can be the care during the pregnancy, both in terms of the detection of possible onset of premature labour and its possible treatment and also the encouragement of greater fetal growth by such measures as rest and improved diet. As stated earlier it should be possible with routine ultrasonic screening to diagnose all, or nearly all, cases of multiple pregnancy before the beginning of the third trimester. In previous publications the percentage of twins diagnosed before delivery has varied from less than 50 per cent up to 94.7 per cent; the figures are

Table 8.1. *Percentage of twins diagnosed before delivery.*

Author	Percentage of twins diagnosed before delivery	Date of study
Farrell	94.7	1957–1963
Robertson	92.0	1956–1962
Spurway	87.8	1946–1958
Law	86.0	1962–1964
Waddell and Hunter	82.3	1949–1959
Jonas	90.0	1954–1961
Tow	80.0	1947–1956
Hallan	69.0	1954–1958
Guttmacher	64.4	1939
Barter	60.0	1965
Danielson	60.0	1940–1957
Kurtz	52.2	1947–1953
Stone and Donnenfeld	< 50.0	1949–1955

shown in Table 8.1. In the North-West London Metropolitan Region Survey (Law, 1967) 86 per cent of the twin pregnancies were diagnosed before the start of labour but the diagnosis was made in only 45.6 per cent before the 32nd week. Thus half of the mothers with a twin pregnancy had progressed undiagnosed beyond the stage when it is usually accepted that extra surveillance and rest should commence. Most reports suggest that a correct diagnosis is eventually made before labour begins in the majority of multiple pregnancies, but the proportion in whom the diagnosis is made in early pregnancy is unexpectedly small.

CHAPTER 9

Management of Multiple Pregnancies

I. MACGILLIVRAY

The perinatal mortality is much higher in multiple pregnancies than in singleton pregnancies and this is also true for morbidity rates (Bender, 1952; Anderson, 1956; Potter, 1963; Myrianthopoulos, 1970; Nylander, 1971a). The higher perinatal mortality and morbidity rates are due to the more frequent occurrence of complications in pregnancy in particular the onset of premature labour and the growth retardation which occurs in many multiple pregnancies. The management of multiple pregnancies, therefore, must be directed towards the prevention, or at least the early detection, of complications and the prevention of premature delivery. Attaining adequate intra-uterine growth is also of great importance.

The management is similar to that for singleton pregnancies but must be more intensive. The earlier that this intensive management can be started the better and early diagnosis is imperative if full advantage of antenatal care is to be taken. As already stated (see Chapter 8) there are good grounds for ultrasonic screening of all patients to make sure of diagnosing the multiple pregnancies as early as is reasonable. Probably ultrasonic scanning between the 16th and 20th weeks will give the optimum number of positive results. Scanning before this time is likely to produce an undue number of false negative results. The diagnosis should, if at all possible, be made by the 20th week of pregnancy. It is not sufficient to rely on picking out the cases where twin pregnancy is suspected by the high weight gain or the undue enlargement of the uterus, because it is in cases where there is poor weight gain in terms of a multiple pregnancy or poor growth of the uterus that it is most important to make the diagnosis.

The amount and type of antenatal care will, to some extent, depend on the time of diagnosis. If the diagnosis is made in early or mid-pregnancy then regular checking at the antenatal clinic will suffice for some weeks, but if the

124

diagnosis is not made until later in pregnancy then it may be necessary to admit the patient immediately to hospital for a much fuller assessment and possibly continued rest. The intensity of the antenatal care will also, to some extent, depend on the number of fetuses present, and again generally speaking the more babies there are the more intensive will be the care and the earlier the admission to hospital.

For singleton pregnancies it is usually recommended that there should be monthly antenatal visits up to the 30th week, fortnightly to the 34th or 36th week and then weekly thereafter. For twin pregnancies the frequency of visits is increased and from 20 weeks they should be seen every three weeks to the 26th week and fortnightly to the 30th week and weekly there-

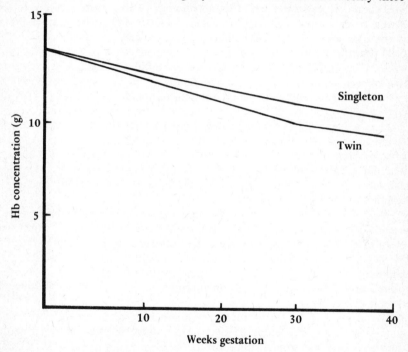

Figure 9.1. Fall in haemoglobin concentration in singleton and twin pregnancies.

after unless they have been admitted to hospital. The frequency of visits will, to some extent, be determined by the distance which the woman has to travel to the clinic, but usually they are quite mobile until 30 weeks. For more multiple pregnancies the patient should be seen weekly and earlier admission to hospital will usually be necessary.

OBSERVATIONS TO BE MADE ANTENATALLY

In addition to the standard observations which are made at the antenatal clinic in all pregnancies it is necessary to make more frequent observations and to make some additional observations in multiple pregnancies. The blood is examined as usual for haemoglobin concentration, but in addition it is highly desirable that the PCV and MCHC should be estimated so that due allowances can be made for the haemodilution which occurs in pregnancy, and more particularly, in multiple pregnancies and which makes the haemoglobin concentration figure more meaningful. The haemoglobin concentration, PCV and MCHC should be estimated at the first visit and again at 30 weeks and thereafter as is considered necessary. In tropical areas where malaria and haemoglobinopathies occur the Hb and PCV are estimated at every visit if facilities exist. The fall in haemoglobin concentration in singleton and twin pregnancies is shown in Figure 9.1. The serum or red cell folate level should be estimated and the morphology of the red blood cells looked at as it is sometimes suggested that megaloblastic anaemia is more common in multiple pregnancies. Although there is no clear evidence of this it is good practice to look at a blood film to see the state of the polymorphonuclear leucocytes and to note any excess lobulation and to estimate the folate level. If there is a microcytic anaemia, as evidenced by a level of haemoglobin concentration which is not accounted for by the fall in PCV and confirmed by a study of the blood film then iron therapy is given. Again if there is a megaloblastic anaemia as evidenced by the blood film and the serum folate levels, then folic acid in a dose of 5 grams per day is given. In some clinics prophylactic iron and/or folic acid is given but it is essential that the same screening for anaemia should be carried out as there is no guarantee that the women are taking the pills. Blood grouping and rhesus testing is done as a routine.

Bacteriological examination of a mid-stream specimen of urine is now usually carried out as a routine in all antenatal clinics, but there is a difference of opinion about whether asymptomatic bacteriuria should be treated or not. Most clinics believe that treatment with a sulphonamide is indicated, or alternatively some give a short course of ampicillin. Others wait until symptoms develop as they believe that unnecessary treatment with antibiotics should be avoided.

The urine must be tested routinely at all visits, not only for protein and glucose but also for acetone. If glycosuria is detected in a random specimen then a second morning fasting specimen of urine is tested with Clinistix and if this is positive it is a strong indication that there is a disturbance of carbohydrate metabolism and a glucose tolerance test should be done (Sutherland, Stowers and MacKenzie, 1970). In pregnancy it is preferable to do an intravenous test as shown by Sutherland and Stowers (1975). In any case it is probably a good thing to do an intravenous glucose tolerance test in all multiple pregnancies because there is a higher incidence of chemical gestational diabetes in twin pregnancies. This is probably due to the higher parity, greater weight and greater incidence of pre-eclampsia in twin than singleton pregnancies. These three factors all predispose to abnormal glucose tolerance in pregnancy. Diabetes is said to be more common in the parents of twins than in those of singletons (Gedda et al, 1969) but further confirmation of this is required.

The blood pressure is recorded carefully as it is most important that a base line of levels is obtained as early in pregnancy as possible for comparison with later levels in view of the high incidence of pre-eclampsia in multiple pregnancies. The blood pressure should be measured with the patient in the left lateral position, particularly in later pregnancy, to avoid the effect of the compression of the large vessels by the uterus causing hypotension.

Weight gain is recorded and charted and if it is below the average for a multiple pregnancy (see Figure 9.2) then this should be taken as evidence of a poor response to pregnancy and careful monitoring of the growth of the babies is required. In some circumstances it is best to admit the patient for rest and observation. If the weight gain is above the average then more frequent observations of the blood pressure and of the urine are required to detect the earliest indications of pre-eclampsia. Neither restriction of the

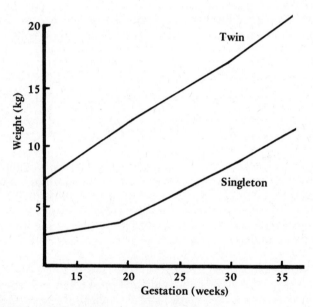

Figure 9.2. Weight gain in singleton and twin pregnancies.

diet nor diuretics should be given to these cases with excessive weight gain as it has been shown by Campbell and MacGillivray (1975) that neither a reducing diet of 1200 calories nor a diuretic reduced the incidence of pre-eclampsia in singletons who had a high weight gain. Furthermore, they showed that the weights of the babies were less than in the control group, so that diuretics or excessive dieting are contraindicated.

The assessment of placental and feto-placental function in multiple pregnancies is very important but it is, of course, difficult to assess the contribution of each fetus or each placenta. Sonar scanning should be carried out to measure the biparietal diameter of the twins, but except where there is marked discrepancy in biparietal diameter there can be difficulty in determining whether the measurements made on each occasion are done on the same biparietal diameters. The ultrasonic method described by Morrison (1974) to measure the weight of the baby may be of considerable value in assessing the growth of twins but still suffers from the problem of identification.

The usual test described for feto-placental function is the estimation of oestriol. It is considered to be a good indicator of feto-placental function because the fetal adrenals convert dehydroisoepiandrosterone sulphate to oestriol. There is some debate about whether the 2×24-hour urine collection is better than a 'spot' plasma sample, but both of course suffer from the deficiency so far as multiple pregnancy is concerned that they give the total value for the two babies and placentas. It is interesting that the oestriol values are about 50 per cent above the singleton values which probably indicates growth retardation in twin pregnancy. Other tests of placental function are human placental lactogen and heat-stable alkaline phosphatase. The plasma volume can also be used as an indicator of the size of the babies as there is a good correlation between plasma volume and baby weight (see Chapter 7).

ADVICE TO WOMEN WITH MULTIPLE PREGNANCIES

REST AND EXERCISE

While it is thought by some that rest encourages growth of the fetus and possibly has a beneficial effect in preventing pre-eclampsia there is the danger, particularly in women with an overdistended uterus, that the pressure of the uterus will predispose to increased risk of thromboembolism. This would also be predisposed to by the changes in the coagulation-fibrinolytic processes in multiple pregnancies. A fine balance has therefore to be drawn in the amount of exercise which should be advocated and the amount of rest which the woman should be advised to take. Towards the end of pregnancy she will become much more clumsy and awkward because of the size of the abdomen and less able to exercise, and it is therefore important that she should have sufficient exercise earlier in the pregnancy. Attendance at a relaxation class should be advocated earlier in pregnancy for these women than for women with singleton pregnancies so that they can take advantage of them before they become too distended. Breathing exercises are of particular importance because of the embarrassment to breathing caused by the diaphragm being pushed upwards.

CLOTHING

Clothing should be loose and non-constrictive but at the same time it is essential that adequate support is given to the over-distended abdomen. This can be achieved with a properly fitted abdominal support.

BATHING

This is no different from the women with singleton pregnancies, but in the later weeks of pregnancy the woman with a multiple pregnancy will probably find it difficult getting in and out of a bath and she may prefer to have a shower or 'wash down' then. In any case she should be assisted in and out of the bath in the later weeks of pregnancy.

SMOKING

As cigarette smoking is known to reduce the weights of babies it is even more important in multiple pregnancies where the babies are likely to suffer from intrauterine growth retardation that the mother is advised not to smoke.

DIET AND DIETARY SUPPLEMENT

Although it is known that starvation causes reduction in baby weight it has, until recently, been suggested that the fetus is a very efficient parasite and that unless the diet is very inadequate the baby weight will not be reduced. This could be a particularly dangerous assumption in multiple pregnancies, and indeed it is possible that lesser degrees of nutritional deficiency can interfere with the baby weight. A recent study in which a 1200 calorie diet was given to primigravidae with a high weight gain caused a reduction in the weights of their babies (Campbell and MacGillivray, 1975). It is difficult to find out from women exactly what they eat but an important observation has been made in non-pregnant subjects and also in pregnant subjects that the 24-hour urinary nitrogen bears a close relationship to the protein intake (Johnstone and MacGillivray, 1975). An estimate of the protein intake can therefore be made in women with multiple pregnancies and supplementation given as required. Alternatively, an arbitrary amount of supplement could be given to all women with multiple pregnancies. It is not known exactly what the requirements are of calories and of protein in pregnancy, but it should be possible to determine this with further studies using the 24-hour urinary nitrogen method. The dietary intake recommended by the World Health Organization for a singleton pregnancy is 2400 kcal and 60 grams of protein, but this is a rather arbitrary figure. For a twin pregnancy the diet should probably be increased to a total of 3000 kcal, but the protein intake probably need not be increased beyond the 60 grams.

BED REST AND HOSPITALISATION

It is generally advocated that women with multiple pregnancies should rest more and there would seem to be at least three potential benefits from this. There is the possibility of avoiding growth retardation, the possibility of reducing the incidence of pre-eclampsia and the possibility of preventing the onset of premature labour. All of these would combine to reduce the peri-natal mortality rate which is between two and four times as great as for single pregnancies (Potter and Fuller, 1949; Guttmacher and Kohl, 1958).

The cause of intrauterine growth retardation in multiple pregnancies is not known, but is possibly related to an inadequate utero-placental perfusion. Measurements of utero-placental blood flow are very difficult to make. The method which is most often quoted is that of clearance of radioactive isotopes and Morris, Osborn and Wright (1955) using radioactive sodium, demon-strated a decrease in the perfusion of the uterus in twin pregnancies compared to single pregnancies of similar gestation. Indirect evidence of reduced perfusion was advanced by Walker and Turnbull (1966) who showed that the cord haemoglobin concentrations were elevated in twins at birth and suggested that this was due to fetal hypoxia. They also found that there was an association between elevated cord haemoglobin levels and infants of below average birthweight.

Although rest in bed is thought to have a beneficial effect on the utero-placental blood supply and is the conventional treatment for pre-eclampsia it has not been proved that rest will increase fetal growth or prevent the onset of pre-eclampsia. Similarly, there has been no real evidence produced to show that rest can prevent the onset of premature labour. If rest increased the utero-placental supply it would be expected that the products of the feto-placental unit would be increased. An increased excretion of oestrogens has been reported in patients on bed rest (Banerjea, 1962; Courey, Stull and Fisher, 1970; Green and Touchstone, 1963) but this was thought by Letch-worth, Howard and Chard (1974) to be due to an increase in the urine volume and they found no increase in the amounts of circulating human placental lactogen.

Many studies have been carried out in the United States and in Britain to try to determine whether rest is effective in preventing any of these complica-tions of twin pregnancies. All of the studies suffer from the fact that none of them was a controlled study. Although such studies have been advocated none has yet been carried out. Another problem is that it would be very difficult to ensure that the women who were not hospitalised were, in fact, not resting. It is quite possible that some of the women who are not admitted to hospital rest more than those who are actually admitted. There are very many other factors concerned with growth retardation, pre-eclampsia and premature labour and all of these would have to be carefully matched in the control group with those who were hospitalised. A further complication is that it is uncertain when strict rest should commence. On the evidence at present available it would seem that if bed rest is thought to be of value it should start around 30 weeks for a twin pregnancy and probably earlier in a triplet or more multiple pregnancy and continue to 37 weeks if the babies are not to be born prematurely, i.e. pre-term. Rest for a shorter period might be beneficial, however, for fetal growth. Hospitalisation of women with multiple pregnancies brings up the difficult question of the economics of this procedure. With hospital costs as they are and the shortage of nursing staff, certainly in the United Kingdom, a hospital stay of seven or eight weeks is very uneconomic. There can also be the added problem of care of existing children in the family and the anxieties created by separation both in them and their mother. The answer probably lies in trying to be selective in the types of patients who are to be admitted for rest and observation and further treatment. This will be referred to later (page 133).

In spite of the inadequacies of the studies which have been carried out to try to determine the benefits of bed rest some of the conclusions are worthwhile considering. Before doing so, however, it is important to emphasise that it is not just bed rest which is involved in hospitalisation; there are other factors which could contribute to reduction in perinatal mortality, growth retardation and pre-eclampsia and prevention of premature labour. In particular, it is quite possible that the nutrition would be improved, certainly in some cases, when the mother is in hospital. The worries and strains of running the home and possibly doing a job are removed, and in general there is a tendency for better results to be obtained when a special interest is taken in a particular condition or complication of pregnancy. It was, of course, no new idea that rest encouraged fetal well-being. This was suggested as early as 1902 by Ballantyne who suggested empirically that rest in the last month of pregnancy would be beneficial. Hirst in 1939 claimed that bed rest, preferably in hospital, from the 36th week onwards encouraged fetal growth and counteracted prematurity and that the average multiple pregnancy could be prolonged to the 38th week.

There were several suggestions in the 1950s (Bender, 1952; Russell, 1952; Anderson, 1956; Tow, 1959) that women with twin pregnancies should be hospitalised for a rest as this would lead to a reduction in the perinatal mortality. They suggested that hospitalisation should start at 30 to 33 weeks and continue for between two and six weeks.

Three reports in 1961 cast doubts on this suggestion. Aaron, Silverman and Halperin (1961) thought it was impractical on the grounds of expense and Bruns and Cooper (1961) did not feel that they could show any evidence to prove or disprove the efficacy of bed rest. Dunn (1961) compared 64 women with twin pregnancies who had no extra rest in bed with 60 women who were rested and found no difference in the perinatal mortality, or the length of gestation and the birthweights were 2495 in the controls and 2581 in the 60 who were rested. In view of the many other factors concerned with birthweight this is not a statistically significant difference and Dunn considered that the effort of hospitalisation was not worthwhile. There then followed a series of reports in the 1960s, most of which claimed some benefit from hospitalisation and rest.

HOSPITALISATION AND PERINATAL MORTALITY

The claims in the 1960s for a reduction in perinatal mortality were advanced by MacDonald (1962) who found a fetal mortality of 8.9 per cent in the rested group (186 cases), compared with 14.6 per cent in the not rested group (314 cases). The groups, however, were not comparable. Brown and Dixon (1963) also claimed a reduction in the perinatal mortality rate, as did Farrel

(1964). As with these other groups Robertson's (1964) was not a controlled study and rest in his cases did not start until the 32nd or 33rd week. He felt that fetal mortality was reduced by rest in bed. The perinatal mortality in Barter's 1965 series of 262 rested twin pregnancies was 10.9 per cent compared with six per cent in 225 controls (Barter, Hsu and Erkenbeck, 1965). In Law's 1962–64 (1967) study there was no alteration in the perinatal mortality. In the most recent study on the effect of bed rest in pregnancy, Jeffrey, Bowes and Delaney (1974) did not find any improvement in perinatal mortality when the cases of less than 36 weeks gestation were excluded. Jonas (1963) found that the perinatal mortality rate was actually higher in the patients rested before the end of the 36th week in primigravidae and there was only a disappointing effect on the perinatal wastage in the multigravidae.

PROLONGATION OF PREGNANCY BY HOSPITALISATION

Most writers who believe that rest in bed reduces the perinatal mortality are agreed that most of the benefit is due to the baby weights being increased and this in turn is due to the prolongation of the pregnancy, although some may be due to better growth of the baby. In 1939 Hirst claimed that bed rest, preferably in hospital, from the 36th week onwards prolonged the average length of multiple pregnancy to 38 weeks. This would counteract prematurity and encourage fetal growth. However, Dunn in 1961 and Jonas in 1963 did not find any evidence of prolongation of pregnancy. This was also found in a most recent study by Jeffrey, Bowes and Delaney in 1974, but Law (1967) thought that there was a slight prolongation of pregnancy.

INCREASED WEIGHTS OF BABIES DUE TO HOSPITALISATION

If, as seems probable, there is no prolongation of pregnancy then the beneficial effect may be on increased growth of the babies. This has mainly been determined by assessing the prematurity rates (babies of less than 2500 grams) in rested groups compared to non-rested groups and a decrease in the prematurity rate was found by Tow in 1959, MacDonald in 1962, Brown and Dixon (1963); in multiparae but not primigravidae by Jonas (1963), by Robertson (1964) and by Barter in 1965. The last author found that there was a difference of 600 grams in the rested compared to the non-rested group. This was by far the greatest difference found by any of the writers. Law found that both first and second twins were heavier in the rested groups. In the most recent study of Jeffrey in 1974 he compared a group in which the twins were not diagnosed until labour or the time of delivery (42 patients), a group in which twins were diagnosed antepartum but no bed rest was used (31 patients), and a third group of 41 patients in which bed rest was used in the management. Bed rest was initiated between 25 and 40 weeks. Most were maintained at bed rest until delivery but a few were allowed normal activity after reaching the 37th week and the duration of bed rest varied from two days to nine weeks. The general policy was to hospitalise for bed rest between the 30th and 37th week of gestation. It is obvious that this study was unsatisfactory in that bed rest was started too late to be meaningful in many cases. There was also no attempt at matching the groups. However, it was concluded that the number of babies who were small for gestational age was less (23.4 per cent) in the bed rest group, compared with 34.6 in the no bed rest group. They were assessed as low for gestational age by the University of Colorado Medical Center classification of newborns by birthweight and gestational age (Battaglia and Lubchenko, 1967).

To summarise, the studies to determine the effects of bed rest and hospitalisation on the outcome of twin pregnancies have all had deficiencies, particularly in standardisation of controls in terms of gestation length, sex of babies, zygosity, placentation, parity, previous obstetric history, age, height, weight, social class, smoking habits and nutrition, and also the time at which rest was started and for how long it was continued. By more careful selection and with large numbers the difficulties would be overcome. On present knowledge, however, it appears that there is little to support the belief that perinatal mortality is reduced by the type and duration of rest which has so far been tried. There is also little to support the belief that the length of pregnancy might be prolonged. However, it would appear that the growth of the baby might be improved and that the baby weights would be increased by bed rest and hospitalisation. To be of real benefit this would have to start at least by 30 weeks and continue until 36 or 37 weeks. Other factors such as improved diet and restriction of smoking might play a part in allowing better growth of the babies. Most of the studies which have been undertaken have suffered from the disadvantage that early diagnosis of the multiple pregnancy was not possible. With the increased possibilities of early diagnosis by ultrasonic screening and the possibility of measuring the content of the diet it should become possible to assess more accurately the effect of rest from an early stage and the effects of good nutrition on baby growth and the outcome of multiple pregnancies.

SELECTION OF PATIENTS FOR HOSPITALISATION AND REST

As previously indicated, it is probably uneconomic as well as possibly unnecessary to hospitalise all patients with multiple pregnancies, but it is advisable to select the high risk groups and insist, as far as possible, on them coming into hospital for rest, observation and possibly increased diet. These high risk cases are the ones most liable to complication of pre-eclampsia, poor intrauterine growth or premature labour. Those with excessively high weight gain or a rise in blood pressure or particularly if they have proteinuria should be admitted early. Those who are found to have any evidence of hyper-irritability of the uterus or more particularly if there is evidence of the cervix effacing or dilating should also be admitted at an early stage.

Probably the ones most likely to benefit are those where there is a risk of poor intrauterine growth of the fetus. This may be indicated by a poor weight gain or by a history of previous small-for-dates babies. Lower social class women are more likely to have smaller babies, particularly if they themselves are small and light. Probably all primigravidas would benefit from hospitalisation because of their greater risk of pre-eclampsia and also because first babies tend to be smaller than subsequent babies. Women of high parity, that is five or more, are also more likely to benefit from hospitalisation.

PREVENTION OF PREMATURE LABOUR

Although in the previous section it was suggested that pregnancy was not prolonged by hospitalisation and rest newer methods of prevention or

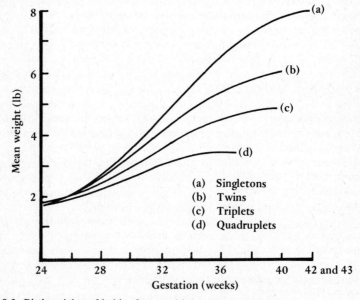

Figure 9.3. Birth weights of babies from multiple pregnancies.

controlling premature labour could be more readily applied while the patient was hospitalised. These are the frequent assessment of the state of the cervix, and the use of beta stimulators to stop uterine activity. Vaginal examinations every two to three days from the 28th week onwards would be likely to determine the early effacement and dilatation of the cervix, particularly in primigravid patients.

The cause of the onset of premature labour in twin pregnancies is not known but it may be due to a disturbance in the balance of hormones, or may be related to uterine distensibility. Many small animals, such as rabbits and guinea pigs, have large litters and have shorter gestation lengths and lower individual birth weights than those with small litters. McKeown and Record (1952) showed that in the human the greater the number of babies the lower the birth weight of each fetus at all gestations from about 30 weeks onwards (see Figure 9.3). However, if uterine distensibility was the only factor involved it would seem likely that apart from cases with hydramnios the combined weights of the babies would be constant, but of course this is not so. McKeown and Record postulated that as gestation progressed the uterus became increasingly sensitive to distension and showed that as the mean combined birth weight increased from 7.53 lb for singletons to 12.28 lb for quadruplets, the mean length of gestation decreased from 280.5 to 236.8 days. These data are compatible with the hypothesis that uterine distensibility is the factor limiting both the length of gestation and the litter weight, but this is far from being proven. Newman (1942) believed that premature labour in twins is due to 'crowding' in the uterus and McKeown and Record suggested that retardation of fetal growth could be attributable to 'crowding' in the uterus. Daw and Walker (1975) confirmed this belief on the basis of underweight women producing lower weight twins and the overweight mothers producing higher weight twins but they admitted that this could simply be related to the smaller woman having a smaller uterus and smaller twins.

USE OF β-ADRENERGIC STIMULATORS AND ETHANOL

β-adrenergic stimulators such as isoxsuprine and ritodrine have been claimed to be of value in stopping premature labour. Their action is local on the smooth muscle of the uterus. They are most effective when given as an intravenous infusion. Ethanol has also been advocated by Fuchs (1965) for the control of uterine activity but unlike the adrenergic stimulators the action of ethanol is central. No control trial has been carried out in multiple pregnancies, but either β-adrenergic stimulators or ethanol can be used.

INCOMPETENCE OF THE INTERNAL CERVICAL OS

Premature labour in the majority of cases of twin pregnancy follows efface-ment and dilatation of the cervix and premature rupture of the membranes follows subsequently in many patients. It would appear that overdistension of the uterus and 'crowding' as described by Newman leads to a sort of physiological cervical incompetence. Barter et al (1963) found that in a large series of patients treated for cervical incompetence none of the patients had had a twin pregnancy previously and none of the patients in the study group of Barter (1965) had premature babies in subsequent singleton gestations. It would appear that the overdistension of the uterus and the stretching of the cervix which occurs in twin pregnancies is a temporary change and does not recur in a subsequent singleton pregnancy.

It is not surprising, therefore, that attempts have been made to prevent premature labour in multiple pregnancies by insertion of cervical sutures, but just as it is difficult to prove the value of cervical sutures in singleton pregnancies, so it has proved equally difficult in multiple pregnancies. Many have tried cervical sutures and a report has been published of this treatment being used even in a triplet pregnancy by Dennerstein (1971). In the case reported by Allahbadia (1962) the patient had had an amputation of the cervix and had premature labour at 28 weeks. This was followed by a twin pregnancy and during this pregnancy the cervix was examined weekly. At 24 weeks the cervix was found to be opening up and a MacDonald (1957) purse-string suture was inserted round the cervix at 24 weeks. The suture was noted to be cutting through the cervical canal at 33 weeks when a second suture was inserted and again at 36 weeks because the previous suture was also cutting in. The patient went into labour spontaneously at 37 weeks. Dennerstein (1971) reviews the 10 cases of cervical ligation performed in twin pregnancies and reported his triplets case. This was in a woman who had spontaneously aborted at 17 weeks in a previous pregnancy and her second and third pregnancies ended in abortion at 10 weeks. Her fourth pregnancy was unsuccessfully treated with a cervical suture and in her fifth pregnancy she had triplets. A cervical suture was inserted at 14 weeks. At 31 weeks there was a spontaneous rupture of the membranes and the babies were delivered and survived. In all of the cases reviewed by Dennerstein there had been an indication other than the multiple pregnancy for inserting the suture. This also applied to the two interesting cases reported by Mc-Gowan (1970). They were twin pregnancies in twin sisters, both of whom had had dilatation of the cervix for dysmenorrhoea and had incompetence of the cervix. Both had unsuccessful pregnancies. McGowan collected information from 18 medical schools on cervical suture (cerclage) in twin pregnancies. There were 43 cases treated mostly with MacDonald's suture with a success rate of 66 per cent. Although it is not stated, presumably they had all had incompetence of the cervix early in pregnancy and the incompetence was not due to the multiple pregnancy.

The use of cervical suture in multiple pregnancies where cervical incompetence is not suspected has not been studied. If, as suggested by Barter, there is a physiological cervical incompetence in twin pregnancies then there would seem to be a strong argument for cerclage in these cases. However, it would be difficult to prove the value of this and the best line of treatment at the moment is probably to do frequent vaginal examinations to assess the state of the cervix and if it should be effacing and dilating to consider inserting a suture then. Probably the MacDonald (1957) type of suture would be the desirable one in such cases as it is unlikely that dilatation of the cervix will be noted until the later weeks of pregnancy when it will be easier to insert the MacDonald suture.

CHAPTER 10

Complications of Twin Pregnancy

P. P. S. NYLANDER AND I. MACGILLIVRAY

It is generally believed that twin pregnancy places a much greater strain on the mother than singleton pregnancy and that for this reason all the complications of pregnancy would occur more frequently in twin pregnancy. In practice, however, only some complications have been found to be particularly associated with multiple pregnancy, others appear to occur just as commonly in twin as in singleton pregnancy. A consideration of the important complications may help to illustrate this.

PRE-ECLAMPSIA

Pre-eclampsia is one of the most important complications in obstetrics, the aetiology of which is still obscure in spite of much research. Some of the difficulties in the study of this condition and in comparing results of different investigators are due to divergence of opinion as to the definition of the condition or the criteria which should be used in classifying the different grades. Nelson (1955) suggested certain diagnostic criteria for grading pre-eclampsia. He defined pre-eclampsia as a condition in which a rise of diastolic blood pressure of 90 mm Hg or more occurred after the 26th week of pregnancy on two or more occasions, separated by at least a day, or in which the rise showed a progressive pattern if the patient was in labour. The pre-eclampsia was classified as mild if there was no albuminuria. If the hypertension was accompanied by definite albuminuria (more than a trace or 0.25 g/litre Esbach) preferably in a catheter specimen of urine, the condition was regarded as severe pre-eclampsia.

The value of these criteria for defining pre-eclampsia were confirmed by a large study in Aberdeen (MacGillivray, 1961). Most investigations have been

137

confined to singleton pregnancies but a few authors have investigated this condition in twin pregnancies as well. Guttmacher (1939a) found that the frequency of pre-eclampsia in viable twin pregnancies was three times that in all viable pregnancies. Bender (1952) also found that this condition occurred about three times as often in twin pregnancies. MacGillivray (1958) has shown that the condition is typically a disease of primigravidae. He found that the incidence of severe pre-eclampsia in primigravidae with twin pregnancies was five times that for singleton pregnancies and even more striking was that in twin pregnancy the incidence of severe pre-eclampsia occurring for the first time in a second pregnancy was 13 per cent compared with one per cent for a singleton pregnancy. These investigators did not distinguish between monozygotic and dizygotic twin pregnancies.

In a recent study conducted in Aberdeen the incidence of severe pre-eclampsia in primigravidae was also found to be much higher in twin maternities than in singleton maternities (the respective figures being 20.3 and 5.1 per cent). The incidence appeared to be higher in monozygotic twin maternities (35.3 per cent) than in dizygotic twin maternities (20.0 per cent) but the difference was not statistically significant (Nylander, 1975, unpublished data).

Pre-eclampsia and eclampsia have also been studied by a few investigators in populations in tropical Africa (e.g., Lawson, 1961; Cannon and Hartfield, 1964; Thompson and Baird, 1967). However, the criteria used for diagnosis in pre-eclampsia in some of these investigations differed from those in the other studies mentioned previously, thus making comparisons difficult. Furthermore, studies appear to have been confined to single pregnancies. In the recent study in Ibadan (Nylander, 1975, unpublished data) however, Nelson's criteria were used for the diagnosis and grading of pre-eclampsia. The incidence of severe pre-eclampsia in pregnancy (for all parities) was found to be 4.5 per cent in twin maternities and 6 per cent in singleton maternities. The incidence in primigravidae was 5.9 per cent for twin maternities and 1.1 per cent for singleton maternities. The incidence appeared to be the same in monozygotic as in dizygotic twin maternities. Pre-eclampsia was found to occur more commonly in labour than in pregnancy. The incidence of severe pre-eclampsia in labour in twin maternities (for all parities) was 7.9 per cent compared with 2.1 per cent for singleton maternities. Again the condition appeared to be as common in monozygotic as in dizygotic twin maternities.

Although the criteria for diagnosis of pre-eclampsia differ in different studies, the diagnosis of eclampsia (convulsions occurring in pregnancy other than epilepsy or other known convulsive states) presents little difficulty. However, this condition occurs relatively rarely and can be prevented by good obstetric care. The study of its incidence is, therefore, difficult because of its rarity and in any case the frequency of this condition is more likely to reflect the standard of obstetric care in the hospital concerned rather than the actual incidence of the disease. In both the recent Aberdeen and Ibadan studies this condition was found to occur more frequently in twin than in singleton maternities. The numbers of maternities involved were too few to compare the incidence in monozygotic and dizygotic twin pregnancies.

The findings from all these studies have indicated the need for special care (routine blood pressure readings and testing of the urine) in mothers expecting twins not only in pregnancy but also in labour so that the onset of pre-eclampsia can be promptly detected and appropriate management commenced. The management of pre-eclampsia and eclampsia in twin pregnancy is the same as in singleton pregnancy. The patient with pre-eclampsia should be admitted for bed rest and sedation in hospital. The use of diuretics and salt restriction is debatable but in view of the findings described in Chapter 9 it is probably advisable to avoid their use. The decision as to the time and mode of delivery will depend on many factors, e.g. the severity of the condition and the size of the babies. The patient with eclampsia should be managed along the usual lines—with anticonvulsants such as chlormethiazole or diazepam, with antihypertensives such as puroverine, diazoxide, or hydrallazine, and epidural anaesthesia.

ANAEMIA

The study of anaemia in pregnancy presents some difficulties because of the varying criteria which may be used in diagnosing the condition. As a result of haemodilution in pregnancy, the PCV or Hb% falls. Difficulty arises in deciding what level should be accepted as normal. In fact, it has been suggested that these indices are not reliable in determining anaemia and that other criteria, e.g. MCHC or serum folate, should be used.

Some studies have been carried out in which the frequency of anaemia (using some of these criteria) has been compared in twin and single pregnancies. Guttmacher (1939a) compared the haemoglobin readings in 1962 single pregnancies with 47 twin pregnancies and found that a much higher proportion of patients with twin pregnancies had a level below 70%. Similar findings have been made in the study of anaemia in patients who were admitted during pregnancy in Aberdeen because their Hb level had fallen below 70% (Nylander, 1975, unpublished data), the incidence of twin maternities being 6.8% compared with 1.1% for singletons. It is, however, likely that the lower Hb level in the twin pregnancies was caused by the greater haemodilution which occurs in twin pregnancy (Rovinsky and Jaffin, 1965; Campbell and MacGillivray, 1972). In the Aberdeen study although the patients included in the analysis were those which had been admitted *solely* because of anaemia, it is probable that patients with twin pregnancies would be more likely to be admitted for anaemia than other patients. This would create a bias which would increase the incidence of the condition in twin maternities. Hall (1970) in her study of folic acid deficiency in pregnancy (using serum folate levels) did not find any evidence of a greater incidence of deficiency in twin pregnancies.

In the study of anaemia in Ibadan (Nylander, 1975, unpublished data), anaemia (PCV < 27%) was found to be just as common in singleton pregnancy as in twin pregnancy, the incidence being 10.6 and 10.4 per cent respectively (Nylander, 1975, unpublished data). This finding is contrary to the general belief that anaemia is more common in twin pregnancy because of the greater demands of the two fetuses on the maternal stores. However, most of the anaemia in this population is due to folic acid deficiency and haemolytic anaemia. For example, Harrison (1969) in his study of anaemia in pregnant women in Ibadan found that 234 (92 per cent) out of 255 women studied had folic acid deficiency anaemia, mostly associated with haemolysis. This haemolytic anaemia is usually due to maternal infection in which the red cells are destroyed directly by the parasites or indirectly by an autoimmune process. This probably accounts for findings of similar incidence in both types of pregnancy since the haemolytic process is likely to affect patients with twin and singleton pregnancies equally. This finding in the Ibadan study is in agreement with that of Hall (1970) in her study of anaemia due to folic acid deficiency in Aberdeen.

The management of anaemia in twin pregnancy is the same as for the condition in singleton pregnancy which includes investigations to determine the cause of the anaemia and treatment with iron, and folic acid, blood transfusion, etc. (depending on its severity). However, in tropical areas where the PCV may fall to very low levels, e.g. below 13 per cent, direct blood transfusion may precipitate cardiac failure because of the greater haemodilution and increased cardiac output which is associated with severe anaemia (particularly in twin pregnancy) and which (in combination with the scarcity of red cells) results in poor oxygenation of the cardiac muscle. Treatment in such cases should be directed to increasing the red cell mass without increasing the blood volume and further overloading the circulation. This can be achieved by a slow transfusion with packed cells and ethacrynic acid (or other fast-acting diuretics). In urgent cases exchange blood transfusion may be required.

HYDRAMNIOS

As in pre-eclampsia and anaemia, the investigation of hydramnios is difficult because of the varying criteria used in its diagnosis. What one observer calls excessive amniotic fluid another may regard as normal. Thus, there is a large subjective element in making the diagnosis depending on clinical impressions of individual observers. This probably accounts for the wide variations reported of the incidence of this condition in pregnancy, i.e. from 0.5 to 24 per cent. The incidence in twin pregnancies reported by McClure (1937), Guttmacher (1939a), Munnell and Taylor (1946), Potter and Fuller (1949), and Bender (1952) were 3.6, 7.0, 5.8, 4.4 and 10.6 per cent respectively. It is noteworthy, however, that in spite of this variation in incidence investigators are generally agreed that hydramnios is more likely to occur in twin pregnancies. It is usually stated that hydramnios (particularly acute hydramnios) is more common in monozygotic twin pregnancy. For example, Gaehtgens (1936) reported a higher incidence of acute hydramnios in single ovum twinning. Guttmacher (1939a) however, reported a fairly similar incidence of hydramnios in monozygotic and dizygotic twin pregnancies.

Since there is so much variation in the criteria used in the diagnosis of hydramnios (as well as variations depending on the subjective impressions of individual observers) it might be felt that the variation in the incidence of this condition in pregnancy reported by different investigators merely reflects variations in methods of diagnosis or in subjective impressions of individual observers. This may be so for singleton pregnancies, but if the frequency of this condition is *several* times higher in twin pregnancy than in singleton pregnancy, then in spite of the variation due to diagnostic criteria, it is likely that a higher incidence will be found in twin pregnancy and this appears to be the case. However, in view of the difficulties of the early investigators in diagnosing zygosity (as mentioned previously) it is unlikely that their reports of incidence in monozygotic and dizygotic twin pregnancies will be reliable.

It was found in both the Aberdeen and Ibadan study that hydramnios is more common in twin than in singleton pregnancy and also that hydramnios was not more common in monozygotic than in dizygotic twin pregnancy as is generally believed (Tables 10.1, 10.2 and 10.3) (Nylander, 1975, unpublished data).

Table 10.1. *Incidence of hydramnios in singleton and twin pregnancy in Aberdeen* (1958–1965).

	Singleton pregnancy	Twin pregnancy
No. of patients with hydramnios	92	7
Total No. of patients	24 178	294
Incidence	0.4%	2.4%

Table 10.2. *The incidence of hydramnios in monozygotic and dizygotic twin pregnancy in Aberdeen.*

	Type of twin pregnancy			
	MZ	DZ	Zygosity not known	All twins
No. of patients with hydramnios	5	16	4	25
Total No. of patients	58	163	73	294
Incidence	8.6%	9.8%	5.5%	8.5%

Table 10.3. *The incidence of hydramnios in singleton and twin pregnancy in U.C.H., Ibadan.*

	Singleton pregnancy	Type of twin pregnancy			
		MZ	DZ	Zygosity not known	All twins
No. of patients with hydramnios	62	2	27	–	29
Total No. of patients	2347	18	129	7	154
Incidence	2.6%	11.1%	20.9%	–	18.8%

It would appear then that there is evidence that hydramnios is more common in twin than in singleton pregnancy and that it is equally common in dizygotic as in monozygotic twin pregnancy.

Since premature labour is very common in twin pregnancy the occurrence of hydramnios may increase the chance of premature labour in such cases. For this reason early detection and management of the condition is important.

The management, as in singleton pregnancy, will include x-ray of the abdomen to exclude fetal abnormality, and bed rest. The use of diuretics is again controversial. Very occasionally, particularly in acute hydramnios, amniocentesis may be required.

ANTEPARTUM HAEMORRHAGE

It is generally believed that the incidence of antepartum haemorrhage is higher in twin pregnancy partly because the larger area of placental attachment is more likely to cause placenta praevia and this type of antepartum haemorrhage. Munnell and Taylor (1946) found a higher incidence of placenta praevia in twin pregnancies. Most recent investigations have, however, failed to show that placenta praevia or antepartum haemorrhage is more common in twin pregnancy. Bender (1952) found an incidence of placenta praevia in twin pregnancy of 0.6 per cent as against 0.9 per cent in singleton pregnancy. Paintin (1962) in his investigation of over 30 000 maternities in Aberdeen found an incidence of 3.0 per cent for antepartum haemorrhage in singleton pregnancies. The incidence in twin pregnancies over the period of study was also 3.0 per cent.

In the recent study of twinning in Aberdeen (Nylander, 1975, unpublished data) out of 45 378 singleton maternities there were 1624 cases of antepartum haemorrhage, an incidence of 3.6 per cent. In twin maternities there were 22 cases out of 567 maternities, an incidence of 3.9 per cent. The incidence in monozygotic twin pregnancy was 3.2 per cent and in dizygotic twin pregnancy, 3.5 per cent. The incidence of antepartum haemorrhage was therefore about the same for both singleton and twin pregnancy and it was equally common in monozygotic and dizygotic twin pregnancy.

The management of antepartum haemorrhage in twin pregnancy is not different from that in singleton pregnancy and depends on the cause of the haemorrhage. X-ray of the abdomen or sonar studies may be able to detect placenta praevia and rest and observation in hospital is indicated until the 37th week when the patient is delivered either by Caesarean section or vaginally following induction, depending on the type of placenta praevia. The mild cases of abruptio placentae can be managed by this expectant method while the severe cases will require immediate active treatment: blood transfusion, induction, correction of fibrinogen depletion if it occurs, vaginal delivery or Caesarean section if necessary.

RHESUS ISOIMMUNISATION

The antenatal management of rhesus isoimmunisation in multiple pregnancy is more complicated than in singleton pregnancies, since it is possible for the babies to be affected to different degrees. Variations in severity may result from differences in rhesus and ABO blood groups, but are not related to the zygosity of the babies (Beischer, Pepperell and Barrie, 1969). The degree of haemolysis can vary even when both fetuses are rhesus-positive, suggesting that factors other than maternal antibody level are involved, and placental permeability to rhesus antibodies may account for some of these differences (Beischer, Pepperell and Barrie, 1969).

If the clinical picture suggests that induction before 37 weeks is not warranted, then management presents little more in the way of problems than for singletons. It is when the disease appears to be more severe that difficulties arise, especially when there is the possibility that one baby may be unaffected, i.e. the father is heterozygous for the rhesus factor. In addition there are the technical difficulties of amniocentesis and intrauterine transfusion. The pregnancy may be managed to give preferential treatment to either the lesser or to the more affected baby but there is no hard and fast practice established. After 36 weeks gestation, with both babies affected, it would be reasonable to induce labour at a time beneficial to the most severely affected baby, but where one is unaffected and the other so badly affected that intrauterine transfusion is indicated, it would seem more logical to continue the pregnancy to as near term as possible in the hope of getting a live healthy baby at the expense of losing one whose chance of survival was poor anyway. In between these two extremes the decision is more difficult, and previous history, gestation, baby size and the hazards of early induction versus intrauterine transfusion must be considered on an individual basis but all twin pregnancies in this group should have an amniocentesis to determine marked differences in haemolysis.

Very little data are available on the detailed management of rhesus incompatibility in twins, and none at all on higher multiples. Valuable information on the severity can be obtained from examination of the liquor amnii but in twin pregnancy there are problems in identifying the individual sac at amniocentesis. Various dyes have been used for identification, e.g. Evan's blue, Coomassie blue (which has the disadvantage that it stains the baby's skin and can cause unnecessary maternal concern) and indocyanine green.

In the past 10 years there have been five sets of rhesus twin pregnancies born in Aberdeen, and three of them required amniocentesis. In one, Evan's blue was the marker, the concentration used was not stated, and in a second case, 2 ml one per cent congo red was injected. In neither of these patients were both sacs entered, and neither had a repeat amniocentesis. In the third case, 4 ml one per cent congo red was injected after withdrawal of liqour, at 30 weeks gestation, but the second sac could not be tapped. It was known that there was an anterior and a posterior placenta, so difficulty in reaching the posterior sac had been anticipated. Two weeks later at repeat amniocentesis, there was enough dye in the liquor to interfere with spectrophotometry, and the dye was still present (though in much lower concentration) and had permeated into the other sac at the time of delivery at 34 weeks. Ellis, Coxon and Noble (1970) found that the indocyanine green injected at intrauterine transfusion had dispersed a week later, but the amount originally instilled in the liquor was not given. In the first of the Aberdeen cases there was no mention of whether or not the liquor was coloured at delivery a week after the procedure, and the second patient aborted only four days after the amniocentesis, and the liquor was pink. The use of dyes would seem to have limited application, especially if they interfere with optical density readings and once they permeate into the other amniotic cavity, they are of no value in identification at repeat examinations. Bowes and Droegemueller (1968) did four amniotic taps, one in each uterine quadrant, but as there was no significant difference in the optical densities of each sample, they concluded

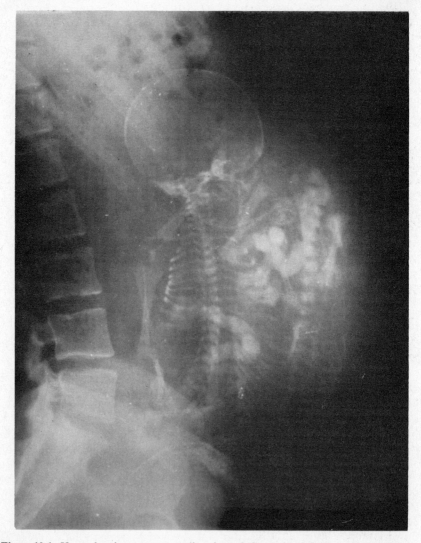

Figure 10.1. X-ray showing contrast medium in each fetus after injection of urografin.

that they had sampled the same cavity on each occasion. They therefore used amniography to outline the extent of one amniotic cavity, and this, together with accurate placental and fetal location by ultrasound would seem to be of value in difficult cases, where repeated taps are anticipated. Amniography is not always necessary, as in the third of the Aberdeen cases, liquor obtained from each side of the uterus (after assessing the fetal position by ultrasound) showed different optical densities, and the fact that both sacs had been entered was confirmed by injecting 60 per cent urografin after each specimen was taken, and x-ray showed the contrast medium had been ingested by each fetus (see Figure 10.1).

INTRAUTERINE INFUSION

In the only completely successful case so far reported (Ellis et al, 1970) each twin received three intraperitoneal transfusions between 27 and 32 weeks gestation. In previous reports one or both babies had died. Fetal position may be assessed either by placing a straight x-ray film over the abdomen, like a map, or by accurate palpation (Ellis et al, 1970) or by means of contrast medium, swallowed by the babies (Crosby and Gheen, 1967; Bowes and Droegemueller, 1968). The procedure itself is no more difficult than it is in singletons, once the babies' positions have been identified. The custom to date has been to transfuse one baby and then the other, but by using a mechanical pump it would seem reasonable to attempt both transfusions simultaneously, making the procedure less time-consuming and more acceptable to the mother.

THREATENED ABORTION

It would be expected that the risk of threatened abortion would be greater in twin pregnancy because two embryos or fetuses are involved. However, the incidence of this complication in the recent Aberdeen study was 3.5 per cent for singleton pregnancies and 3.9 per cent for twin pregnancies. The incidence in monozygotic twin pregnancy was 3.2 per cent and in dizygotic twin pregnancy it was the same (3.2 per cent).

There was therefore no significant difference in the frequency of threatened abortion in twin and singleton pregnancy. The complication was equally common in monozygotic and dizygotic twin pregnancy.

COMBINED INTRAUTERINE AND EXTRAUTERINE PREGNANCIES

The incidence of such combined pregnancies has been estimated to be between one in 12 000 and one in 30 000 pregnancies by Winer, Bergman and Fields (1957). Failure to diagnose can have a serious effect either on the intrauterine pregnancy or the extrauterine pregnancy. The intrauterine pregnancy may be diagnosed and the extrauterine pregnancy missed or vice versa. Usually, however, it is the ectopic pregnancy which is removed and there is failure to recognise that there is an intrauterine gestation also present. The viable intrauterine pregnancy may be destroyed by a curettage. If the intrauterine pregnancy is recognised the chances of a progressing pregnancy can be improved by suitable postoperative therapy following the laparotomy for the ectopic pregnancy.

OTHER COMPLICATIONS

There is no evidence that any of the other complications such as pyelitis, hyperemesis gravidarum, heartburn, etc. occur more frequently in twin pregnancy. Guttmacher (1939a) and Bender (1952) found that hyperemesis was not a significant feature of twin pregnancy. Guttmacher (1939a) in his investigation of pyelitis of pregnancy was astonished at the low incidence in twin pregnancy in view of the greater pressure on the ureters which would be expected in twin pregnancy.

The management of these complications is along the same lines as for singleton pregnancies.

CHAPTER 11

Labour in Multiple Pregnancies

I. MACGILLIVRAY

Labour is particularly hazardous in multiple pregnancies, not only because labour tends to occur prematurely but also because of the malpositions and malpresentations which are likely to be present. The prognosis for the babies is likely to be improved the earlier the diagnosis is made in pregnancy and there is a serious risk to the babies if the diagnosis is not made until delivery is being undertaken and especially if the diagnosis is not made until after the first baby is born and ergometrine has been given. Early diagnosis, care during pregnancy and the prevention of the onset of premature labour are therefore vitally important.

ONSET OF LABOUR

The cause of the onset of normal labour is not yet fully elucidated and the reasons for the greater tendency for premature labour to occur in multiple pregnancies is therefore not established. Factors which are likely to contribute are the over-distension of the uterus and the increased production of hormones. Over-distensibility of the uterus is not, however, the only, or even the major cause, of the onset of labour as it would be likely then that the combined weights of the baby would only equal the average weight of a single baby born at term.

Premature labour is by definition the onset of labour before 37 weeks, that is pre-term. The length of gestation is shorter in twin pregnancies than in singletons, averaging about 260 days (see Table 11.1). In the British Perinatal Mortality Survey there were 29 per cent of pre-term deliveries among like-sexed twins and 17 per cent amongst unlike-sexed twins. The mean length of gestation of the twins of like sex was 262 days, which was

Table 11.1. *Length of gestation in twin pregnancies.*

Author	Gestation length	Like male	Like female	Unlike
McKeown and Record (1952)	days	261.8	260.9	262.2
Karn (1952)	days	256.96	256.96	257.43
Guttmacher and Kohl (1958)	weeks	37.1	37.2	36.2
British Perinatal Mortality Survey (1958)	days	262.0	262.0	268.3

significantly less than that of twins of unlike sex at 268.3 days. In other reported series (Table 11.1) however, the difference has not been found to be significant. It seems unlikely that the sex of the baby would determine the onset of premature labour.

Although there is a much fuller understanding of the initiation of labour in the sheep following the elegant work of Liggins, Kennedy and Holm (1967) there is still considerable doubt about whether the same processes occur in the human. These workers have shown that the fetal pituitary and adrenal play an important role in initiating labour in the sheep in which the probable pattern is that the fetal pituitary exerts an influence on the adrenal from which dehydroisoandrosterone is produced. This is the main precursor for oestriol which increases the sensitivity of the myometrium to oxytocin. According to Csapo (1961) progesterone dominance of the myometrium is the important factor in initiating labour. Although there are intermittent so-called Braxton–Hicks contractions occurring throughout pregnancy these contractions do not become regular until labour begins. Probably more important, however, is the occurrence of retraction along with contractions in labour and we do not know what it is that initiates the retractions. During pregnancy the myometrium is fairly insensitive to oxytocin and it is not until nearer term that there is increasing sensitivity. It is not clear, however, what it is that prevents the activity of oxytocin on the myometrium or desensitises the myometrium.

In a review of the initiation of labour Robinson and Thorburn (1974) concluded that the fetus probably initiates labour in the human as in other species but the activation of the anterior pituitary/adrenal system in the human fetus is not as dramatic as in the fetal lamb. Present evidence favours the view that glucocorticoids play a role in initiation of labour in the human. They quote Tamby Raja, Anderson and Turnbull (1974) as showing an increase in 17β-oestradiol preceding the onset of premature labour in the human. This increase in oestradiol could cause a parallel increase in the myometrial biosynthesis of prostaglandin which is responsible for uterine activity in the last two months of pregnancy and this in turn would cause gradual effacement of the cervix.

The state of the cervix has also been studied in relation to the onset of labour and Wood and co-workers (1965) found, by assessing the cervical and myometrial activity from 24 weeks until delivery, that neither alone gave rise to premature labour, but these two factors in combination were likely to do so.

There have been no reported studies on either the endocrine balance or the state of the cervix in relation to the onset of premature labour in twin pregnancies. In view of the great importance of premature labour in multiple pregnancies it would seem that studies of the hormonal balance, the uterine activity and the state of the cervix would be very important and helpful in managing twin pregnancies and preventing or counteracting premature labour.

PROCESS OF LABOUR

Like all other smooth muscle the myometrium undergoes spontaneous activity even when denervated. It is thought that in normal labour there is an area of pacemaker activity in the region of the cornua. Induction of labour by oxytocins might in theory be improved by the administration of oestrogens, but this has not been found in practice. Withdrawal of the progesterone block causes increased oxytocin sensitivity, but in the human it has not been possible to delay the onset of spontaneous labour by giving progesterone or synthetic progestogens in large doses. The level of oxytocinase is increased during pregnancy and it is possible that this is to prevent stimulation of the uterus prematurely, but labour does not seem to occur any more readily in patients with low oxytocinase levels.

The state of the cervix in relation to the onset of premature labour seems particularly important in twin pregnancies as it is possible to detect changes by frequent vaginal examinations. Chemical changes in the collagen fibres and the water content of the cervix and changes in the microscopic architecture of the cervix have been shown in animals before the onset of labour. There is an increase in the ground substance and a loosening of the collagen. These changes may be under control of hormones, particularly oestriol, but they have not so far been correlated with hormone changes in the human.

Softening, effacement and dilatation of the cervix indicate ripeness and these changes tend to occur in women who are likely to go into premature labour and it should be possible to attempt to stop the onset of premature labour (see Chapter 10).

LENGTH OF LABOUR IN MULTIPLE PREGNANCY

As accelerated labour has become more fashionable reliance has to be placed on older reports to determine the length of natural labour in multiple pregnancies. Bender in 1952 found no significant difference in the length of labour in twin compared to singleton pregnancies. Ross and Philpott (1953) found that in 183 twin pregnancies the average length of labour among the 129 multiparae was 8 hours 18 minutes and there were no cases of prolonged labour. Among the 55 primiparae there were four cases of prolonged labour, i.e., 48 hours or longer, and the average duration of the remainder was 12 hours 42 minutes. Law (1967) found that in 954 cases the first stage of labour was completed in under 12 hours in 75.6 per cent of all uncomplicated cases. In 20.1 per cent of primiparae and 3.4 per cent of multiparae the first stage was prolonged beyond 24 hours. In primiparae the second stage of labour lasted between 30 and 120 minutes and in multiparae between 30 and 60 minutes. The second stage was prolonged over two hours in 6.8 per cent of patients. Law suggested that in relation to the perinatal mortality the duration of the second stage should be between 60 and 120 minutes from the point of view of both infants.

EFFECT ON THE MOTHER

Labour in the mother with a multiple pregnancy is more likely to be more disturbing and distressing and indeed exhausting than for the mother of a singleton. This is not necessarily because of any greater pain from uterine contractions but from the fact that with the over-distension and weight of the uterus the general discomfort is greater.

The relief of pain during labour is important particularly in view of the greater general discomfort from which the patients with multiple pregnancies are liable to suffer. Pain can be relieved in the conventional ways with analgesics, such as pethidine, or by epidural analgesia. The advantages of epidural analgesia in the continuous form are the complete freedom from pain and the possibility of performing various manipulations during the second stage of labour. While it is claimed by some that in twin delivery epidural analgesia should not be used because the desire to bear down is removed, others believe that epidural analgesia is indicated for twin delivery because the urge to bear down before full dilatation of the cervix is abolished and the obstetrician can have better control of an assisted delivery. The mother is also more cooperative that when under an inhalational analgesic.

The fluid and food intake should be carefully regulated during labour and it is particularly important that acetonuria should be avoided. In many cases it is necessary to give a glucose infusion. At the same time it is important to avoid giving food by mouth in case a general anaesthetic is required. The usual practice is to avoid giving solid food and to give an alkaline mixture, such as 15 ml of magnesium trisilicate mixture every two hours during established labour. It is important that if at all possible a skilled obstetric anaesthetist should be present for a multiple delivery whether this is undertaken with epidural or when a general anaesthetic might be necessary.

Experimental studies done under epidural analgesia (Lees, Scott and Kerr, 1970) showed there was a marked increase in the left ventricular work of the heart. The cardiac output rose by some 25 per cent with contractions due to a rise in the stroke volume and without any rise in heart rate and the arterial blood pressure rose by about 10 mm Hg. These measurements were made in women with singleton pregnancies and as it is known that the blood volume is greater in multiple pregnancies presumably cardiac output is also greater and there is an even more marked effect in labour. This might have some effect when there is the sudden release of caval pressure and a greatly increased return to the heart when the woman is delivered in the lithotomy position.

The dangers of over-breathing are also important in multiple pregnancies because the maternal Po_2 and pH rise and the maternal Pco_2 may fall to very low levels. This, in theory, could affect the fetal arterial Po_2 but it is unlikely that even in a multiple pregnancy labour the low maternal Pco_2 would last for very long, particularly if it did not arise until the second stage of labour.

EFFECTS ON THE FETUSES

UTERO-PLACENTAL BLOOD SUPPLY

During contractions, particularly if the woman is lying on her back, there is compression of the inferior vena cava and the pelvic veins and the common iliac arteries by the uterus. Unless maternal hypotension is produced, however, this compression is unlikely to be a hazard to the fetuses. However, it is advisable to nurse the woman on her left side during labour.

If the fetal arterial blood pH is maintained at a reasonable level the fetus will survive. There is a redistribution of the fetal blood flow when there is a deterioration in fetal oxygen levels so that the umbilical flow is maintained and the pulmonary and femoral flows may be reduced. The flow to the coronary and cerebral vessels is improved and thus the supply of glucose to the heart and brain is improved.

The changes in the fetal blood gases, that is the Po_2 and the Pco_2, in labour can be measured by means of fetal scalp sampling, but this, of course, is only applicable to a singleton pregnancy and the condition of both babies in a twin pregnancy can only be studied by fetal heart monitoring, or, as has been suggested more recently, by fetal encephalographic studies, or even fetal respiratory studies.

The behaviour of the fetal heart in labour has been studied intensively in recent years and the patterns of behaviour in different circumstances of fetal distress are now quite well understood. The first sign of lowered fetal oxygenation is a fetal tachycardia with a rise to 160 beats per minute or more. Fetal bradycardia involves a dip from the normal 140 beats per minute to 100 beats per minute or less which synchronises with uterine contraction and recovery of the original rate occurs as the contraction passes off (type I dips are thought to be due to higher pressure on the fetal head or intermittent pressure on the cord) and the fetal scalp pH is unchanged. On the other hand, type II dips, that is bradycardia which persists for one or more minutes after the contraction has disappeared, are of serious significance and indicate some degree of myocardial anoxia in the baby.

The passage of meconium is generally considered to be an indication of fetal distress, but of course in a multiple pregnancy it will only be the liquor from the first sac which will show meconium staining.

EFFECT OF DIFFICULT LABOURS

Problems with delivery of the babies of a multiple pregnancy are likely to arise and this is due very often to the malpresentations and malpositions which occur. There have been several reports on the ways in which twins present. Most authors are agreed that both babies present by the vertex in about 45 per cent of cases (see Table 11.2).

Table 11.2. *Vertex presentations in twin pregnancies.*

Author	Percentage presenting both as vertex
Potter and Crunden (1941)	47.8
Portes and Granjon (1946)	44.3
Potter and Fuller (1949)	44.1
Guttmacher and Kohl (1958)	46.9
Zuckerman and Brzezinski (1961)	46.3
Law (1967)	44.1

The presentations of twins have been recorded by Guttmacher and Kohl (1958). In 411 viable twins they found 46.9 per cent were both vertex, 37 per cent—one as a vertex and the other as a breech, 8.7 per cent both breech, 4.9 per cent—one transverse and one vertex, 1.9 per cent—one transverse and one breech, and in 0.6 per cent both were transverse. Portes and Granjon (1946) found that the corresponding figures were 44.3, 38.4, 9.9, 5.3, 1.4 and 0.2 per cent. The incidence of cephalic presentations for all the twins was 66.3 per cent. For the first twin it was 74.9 per cent and for the second twin it was 57.7 per cent. Ross and Philpott (1953) found in 55 primiparae both vertex 34.5 per cent, first vertex, second breech 30.9 per cent, first breech, second vertex 5.5 per cent, both breeches 14.5 per cent, compound 10.9 per cent, brow (first or second) 1.7 per cent, face 1.7 per cent, transverse lie second 0, miscellaneous 0, and in 129 multiparae the corresponding figures were 37.1, 33.1, 12.4, 7.4, 4.1, 2.5, 0, 2.4, 0.8 (first face and prolapse cord, second breech). In the British Perinatal Mortality Survey the method of delivery is shown in Table 11.3.

Table 11.3. *Method of delivery in the British Perinatal Mortality Survey, 1958.*

Method of delivery	Percentage distribution		
	Twin 1	Twin 2	Singletons
Spontaneous vertex			
occipito-anterior	63.6	40.8	85.4
occipito-posterior	3.4	7.3	2.4
Forceps	7.8	7.8	4.7
Assisted breech	18.9	34.0	2.1
Internal version	0.5	4.3	0.1
Caesarean section	3.9	3.9	2.7
Remainder	1.9	1.9	2.6
Total number equal to 100%	206	206	16 994

It should be noted that the excess of breech deliveries in their series of twins was not limited to the pre-term deliveries. In babies delivered at

37 weeks or more 21 per cent of first-born twins and 34 per cent of second-born twins were delivered by the breech, whilst this occurred in only two per cent of singleton deliveries. Breech deliveries and internal versions and forceps deliveries are obviously potentially more traumatic to the fetus than are spontaneous deliveries, and as internal versions and breech deliveries are more common in the second twin this probably accounts for at least part of the higher mortality rate in second twins.

RELATIVE RISKS TO FIRST AND SECOND TWINS

Almost all recent surveys (Donnelly, 1956; Corston, 1957; Little and Friedman, 1958; Guttmacher and Kohl, 1958; Tow, 1959; Danielson, 1960; MacDonald, 1962; Spurway, 1962; Robertson, 1964; Ferguson, 1964; Law, 1967; Patten, 1970) are agreed that there is a higher perinatal mortality for the second twin than for the first (see Chapter 14).

The dangers to the two babies are different in that prolapse of the cord is the major risk to the first baby and malpresentations to the second baby. MacDonald (1962) for example, found that prolapse of the cord occurred ten times with the first twin, causing four deaths and seven times with the second twin but without loss. Breech presentation with breech extraction and compound presentation with internal version are more often required for the second child. Although intervention is more often required for the delivery of the second twin, it is not necessarily the operative manipulations which cause the death but rather the asphyxia associated with the mal-presentation, the reduced placental circulation and sometimes placental separation. Indeed, without intervention the death rate would be higher.

The Apgar score was used by Ware (1971) to assess the risks to the twins. There was a higher incidence of fair or poor Apgar scores in second twins compared with first twins, particularly when delivered by total breech extraction or version and extraction. Birth asphyxia was also studied by MacDonald (1962) in 140 cases where delivery of both babies was by the vertex and it was found that the second twin was more often severely asphyxiated than the first.

INTERVAL BETWEEN BIRTH OF FIRST AND SECOND TWINS

As shown by Wood and Pinkerton (1966) the intra-amniotic pressure after the delivery of the first twin can be altered by several factors. The pressure will tend to be increased by the reduction of the uterine volume and the coincident shortening of the muscle fibres will tend to decrease the force of myometrial contractions. The intra-amniotic pressure may also be influenced by an increase in the production of endogenous oxytocin when the first twin is delivered. They recorded uterine activity in three patients before and after delivery of the first twin in order to study the effect of the sudden and large alteration of uterine volume upon uterine function. Uterine activity continued immediately after the delivery of the first twin as happens in similar experiments on the rabbit uterus. Greenhill (1955) had advocated waiting for an hour before rupturing the membranes but in 1960 he reduced this to 15 minutes. MacDonald (1962) advocated rupturing the membranes of the second sac five minutes after delivery of the first twin. If spontaneous delivery does not occur in 10 minutes after rupturing the membranes, or if any complication arises, operative delivery is indicated. Delivery should thus be complete within 20 minutes of the birth of the first child. He found that operative intervention was required only twice for the second child after a spontaneous first delivery and concluded that early rupture of the membranes of the second sac was not associated with inertia and indeed, the risk of complications seemed to be reduced.

Reports of the second twin being retained for an abnormally long time are rare nowadays apart from those coming from developing countries. Adeleye (1972), reporting recently from Nigeria on 106 cases of retained second twin between 1964 and 1968, again showed that the perinatal mortality rate of a second twin was higher than that of a first twin and the mortality was related to the length of time that the twin was retained. Malpresentation and uterine inertia were the main causes of the retention. He defined retained as being more than 30 minutes, but unfortunately, he does not record the actual length of time that the second twin was retained. Presumably some of them must have been retained for several hours as 55 out of a total of 106 cases of retained second twin were emergency admissions having been delivered of the first twin outside the hospital. The perinatal mortality in the hospital-delivered group was 23.5 per cent compared with 50.4 per cent in the emergency admission group. Williams and Cummings (1953) reported the delivery of twins 56 days apart from a woman with a uterus didelphys. In a similar case Dorgan and Clarke (1956) reported that the babies were born at 31 and 34 weeks gestation respectively. Although it was commonly believed that the delivery of twins some days apart could only occur in malformed uteruses there have been cases confirmed by hysterosalpingography where the uterus was found to be quite normal (Abrams, 1957; Drucker, Finkel and Savel, 1960) and no explanation has been advanced to account for these cases.

DIFFICULTIES IN TWIN DELIVERIES

Difficulties and/or dystocia in multiple pregnancies occur frequently partly because of the malpositions and malpresentations, but also because of the over-distension of the uterus interfering with uterine activity. Although, as stated earlier, the length of the first stage of labour is not prolonged in a multiple pregnancy compared to a singleton this does not necessarily imply that the uterus is acting just as efficiently. Eastman (1961) postulated that in twin pregnancies the amount of cervical dilatation before labour commences is often considerable and that the uterine activity during the labour must be less than in a singleton in order that the total length of labour is the same as in the singleton labour. It was shown by Garrett (1960) that the average duration of labour in 100 matched pairs of twin and singleton pregnancies was the same. Evidence was advanced to support this hypothesis by Friedman and Sachtleben (1964). They measured the rate of cervical dilatation in primigravid and multiparous twins and singleton pregnancies and found that there was a longer latent phase in singleton pregnancies than in multiple pregnancies and a tendency to lengthening of the active phase in twin pregnancies. The latent phase has been described by Friedman (1954) as the interval when the cervix is undergoing softening and effacement preparatory to dilatation and the active phase is the term for dilatation of the cervix. They also found that there was a significantly greater amount of cervical dilatation before labour in the twin pregnancies and this gave rise to the clearly defined shortening of the latent phase. The uterine over-distension apparently resulted in a prolongation of the active phase so that the total duration of labour was within the normal range for singletons.

As in singleton pregnancies factors such as maternal age, parity, stimulation with oxytocics, amount of sedatives and analgesics, the amount of cephalo-pelvic disproportion and the weight of the presenting infant may have an effect on the course of labour. When 50 twin and 50 singleton labours were matched for these factors, Friedman and Sachtleben (1964) did not find any difference in the pattern of labour between the two groups. Some of these factors are more likely to occur in twin pregnancy, such as advanced maternal age and possibly more analgesics being given, but to compensate for this the infant's weight is less. However, the infant's position is more likely to be abnormal in the twin labour. On theoretical grounds, taking into account the over-distension of the uterus and the more frequent occurrence of malpositions and malpresentations, it is surprising that the overall length of labour is the same in singletons as in twins and can only be accounted for by the preliminary dilatation of the cervix which occurs. Presumably the malpositions and malpresentations are compensated for by the smaller size of the twin which is presenting.

Although the first stage of twin labour is not longer than that of a singleton the second stage of labour is only of the same length because it is so often necessary to expedite it because of malposition or malpresentation of the babies and also, of course, because a greater length of time would have to be allowed for the delivery of both babies.

MANAGEMENT OF LABOUR

At the onset of labour in a multiple pregnancy it is essential to carry out a vaginal examination to determine the presenting part and to exclude cord presentation or prolapse. Although it is unlikely in twin pregnancy because of the smaller size of the baby that a cephalo-pelvic disproportion will occur, nevertheless, it is essential to exclude contraction of the pelvis at this examination if this has not already been done during pregnancy. The progress of labour must be carefully assessed and this can be done on a partograph as described by Philpott which incorporates a record of cervical dilatation as described by Friedman (1954). A partogram is shown in Figure 11.1 for a twin pregnancy. The strength, frequency and duration of uterine contractions are

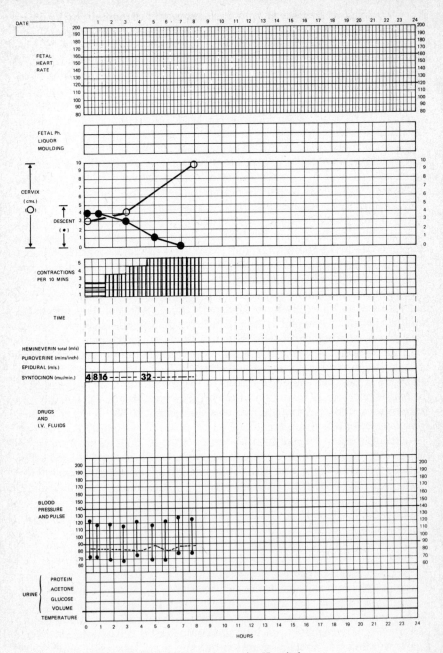

Figure 11.1. Partogram used in Aberdeen Maternity Hospital.

recorded. Where the facilities exist this may be done with a tocograph. Recordings of the fetal hearts are also made, for example, with an electrode attached through the cervix to the presenting part of the first baby and an external Doppler instrument for the second twin. If induction has been performed by rupture of the forewaters it is probably better to leave only a short interval of time before setting up a syntocinon infusion.

There is some controversy about the use of epidural analgesia for relief of pain in labour in twin pregnancies, but this is probably preferable to analgesics such as pethidine or the use of nitrous oxide and oxygen. In any case efficient relief of pain is essential.

A decision about a Caesarean section should be taken preferably before the onset of labour. Generally speaking if any difficulty or delay is anticipated in a twin labour it is better to do an elective Caesarean section. These difficulties may arise because of malpresentations of the baby and this will be dealt with later. Caesarean section may be indicated for complications such as severe pre-eclampsia or ante-partum haemorrhage or in the older primigravida. Previous Caesarean section, depending on the indications for this, may be a reason for repeating the Caesarean section. Caesarean section may occasionally be necessary for the second twin in cases of unsuspected disproportion.

Because of the frequency of malpresentations cord prolapse may occur. It is important, therefore, to do a vaginal examination when the patient goes into labour and also when the membranes rupture. If the cervix is not sufficiently dilated for immediate vaginal delivery a Caesarean section should be carried out in cases of cord prolapse.

During labour the usual observations are made and it is important that fluids are given if necessary intravenously. The patient should be nursed on her left side as far as possible.

When the second stage is reached unless there is some contraindication the patient is encouraged to bear down and an episiotomy should always be performed. This can be done under the epidural anaesthesia or if this has not been performed a perineal infiltration or pudendal block is done.

The delivery of the twins can be completely spontaneous. If the first twin is presenting as an occipito-anterior or a direct occipito-posterior or even as a mento-anterior it can be anticipated that it will be delivered spontaneously by the mother's own efforts. After the delivery of the first twin the lie and presentation of the second twin is determined by abdominal palpation.

If the first twin is in a longitudinal lie and presenting by the vertex the membranes of the second sac should be ruptured without delay. At vaginal examination the presentation is confirmed before rupturing the second sac. It used to be considered that the uterus should be allowed to recover after the delivery of the first twin and to allow an interval of half an hour to elapse before rupturing the second membranes, but this might allow the cervix to close. In most cases the uterus will be active and delivery will take place, but it may be necessary to assist with forceps or ventouse.

When the second baby is presenting by the breech the membranes are ruptured and this should again be done promptly because it is important that the cervix should not close down and possibly interfere with the delivery of the head. The woman is encouraged to bear down, but although a spontaneous breech delivery can occur it is likely that some assistance will be required, particularly with the delivery of the after-coming head. This is preferably carried out with forceps, but if there is any delay in the head coming into the pelvis the Mauriceau–Smellie–Veit manoeuvre can be employed to bring the head down in the transverse position through the brim of the pelvis and into the cavity. It is unlikely to be necessary, however, because with the delivery of the shoulders, again preferably by the Lovsett manoeuvre, the head will generally come into the pelvis. However, if it is caught in the cervix it may be necessary to use the Mauriceau–Smellie–Veit manoeuvre.

ASSISTED DELIVERY OF THE FIRST TWIN

This may be necessary if there is a malposition or malpresentation or if there is uterine dysfunction. The appropriate procedure is carried out. In the case of a transverse lie or a brow presentation Caesarean section will be indicated unless the baby is very small and the brow will turn down through the pelvis. Delay with an occipito-anterior position is dealt with by application of forceps, or, if preferred, the ventouse. Occipito-posterior position may be dealt with either by forceps extraction in the occipito-posterior position or by rotation, either manually or with Kielland's forceps, and delivery in the occipito-anterior position. With a twin pregnancy it is preferable to deliver in the occipito-posterior because the baby is usually small and rotation of the trunk may be difficult because of the presence of the second twin. Occipito-transverse positions are dealt with either by manual rotation or Kielland's forceps. Mento-anterior positions can be dealt with by forceps extraction but mento-posterior positions will require either correction or, if there is relative disproportion, Caesarean section. If it is a breech presentation a full breech extraction may be required if there is uterine dysfunction and the patient is unable to bear down sufficiently. It is, however, more likely that part of the baby will be delivered and an assisted delivery will be carried out.

In cases of contracted pelvis of mild degree it is difficult in a primigravid twin labour to determine whether there will be cephalo-pelvic disproportion, particularly with the second twin, if the pregnancy is at or near to term. Mild contraction of the pelvis is an indication for Caesarean section in a twin pregnancy at, or near, term if the babies are considered to be of average or above average size and particularly if one or both are breech presentations. The weights of previous babies will be a guide in parous women. Caesarean section may be necessary after vaginal delivery of the first twin if the second twin is much larger than the first.

Generally speaking, in most twin deliveries it should be possible to deliver the first baby either under epidural or pudendal block analgesia. If a general anaesthetic is required then, of course, the second twin should be delivered while the patient is still under the general anaesthetic and this is accomplished either by forceps, ventouse or breech extraction. If it is done under an epidural or pudendal block the labour is proceeded with as though the first twin had been delivered spontaneously.

DELIVERY OF THE SECOND TWIN

There have been many reports on the problems of the delivery of the second of twins and the risks to which it is subjected. Most have suggested that the prognosis for the second twin is less favourable than the first, but opinion is by no means unanimous (see Chapter 14). Breech presentation, breech extraction, compound presentation and internal version are all more common for the second child so that the need for operative intervention is greater than for the first twin.

Delivery of the second twin should be carried out early and in a controlled fashion. The membranes of the second sac are ruptured within five minutes of delivery of the first baby after checking that the second baby is in a longitudinal lie. The head or breech should be pushed into the pelvis before rupturing the membranes. It is preferable that during labour an infusion should be set up containing 0.5 unit of syntocinon in 450 ml of dextrose. This can either be infused during the first stage and during the delivery of the first twin if necessary, or alternatively, the infusion can be running on dextrose alone and if there is delay in the uterus contracting after delivery of the first twin the syntocinon infusion is switched on at 15 drops per minute. If the head remains high it is preferably brought down with the ventouse or an internal version can be performed followed by a breech extraction. In most cases this should not be necessary if the syntocinon infusion is running in when the head can be expected to come down far enough into the cavity of the pelvis to allow a forceps extraction. Similarly, if the breech is presenting an assisted breech delivery, or breech extraction, can be performed. However, if a general anaesthetic has been given internal version and breech extraction may be more often required and this in turn will raise the perinatal mortality risk. This is why many advocate epidural or pudendal block in preference to general anaesthesia.

Operative intervention is more often required for the second twin and preferably this should be with forceps or ventouse in cephalic presentations and internal version should be avoided if possible.

The greatest problems arise when the second twin is lying transversely and the membranes rupture before the lie can be corrected. This may occur if the twin pregnancy is not diagnosed until after delivery of the first twin, or in the rare cases of monoamniotic twins, or when the first twin is born without a skilled attendant being present.

In such cases there is a danger of asphyxia because of interference with the placental circulation, or partial placental separation. The liquor will have drained away, the cord may have prolapsed and the uterus may be tightly wrapped around the baby. If this has not yet happened it may be possible to do an internal version and breech extraction but a careful assessment under general anaesthesia must be performed. Should it be thought that there will be difficulty in doing this then it is preferable to perform a Caesarean section both for the sake of the mother and the baby. In some cases the baby will have died and it will be necessary to perform a decapitation.

Occasionally heavy bleeding occurs after the delivery of the first twin and as it is uncertain whether this is coming from the placenta of the second twin the delivery must be completed as expeditiously as possible.

When there has been a long interval since the delivery of the first twin the cervix will probably have closed down and in such cases after checking that the lie of the second twin is longitudinal the membranes are ruptured if they are still intact and an infusion of syntocinon is set up.

When a twin pregnancy has not been diagnosed and an oxytocic such as ergometrine or syntometrine has been given with the delivery of the first baby the second twin is obviously at grave risk and should be delivered as expeditiously as possible. As soon as it is recognised that there is a second baby present the membranes should be ruptured after correcting the lie if necessary and the second baby delivered. It may be necessary in such cases to give a general anaesthetic if the cervix has closed down. Halothane may be necessary to cause relaxation of the uterus to allow extraction of the second twin. If the second twin has died it is still preferable to deliver the second twin fairly expeditiously.

LOCKED TWINS

This is an extremely rare complication of twin labours and is said to occur in about one in 90 000 deliveries or approximately one in 1000 twin births. In the classical type of locked twins the first twin presents by the breech and the second by the vertex and there is chin-to-chin locking of the two heads (Figure 11.2). Another type of entanglement of twins causing dystocia is termed collision, in which delivery of one twin is obstructed by some parts of the other twin, for example, two heads (Figure 11.3) or two breeches trying to get into the pelvis simultaneously or the aftercoming head of the twin in a breech presentation being caught by the trunk of the second twin which is lying in a transverse position. Twins in collision are usually considered together under the generic term of twin-locking. There have been several reviews of literature on twin-locking. One of the most extensive was that of Nissen in 1958 who reviewed the literature from 1882 to 1957 and found 69 cases and added another. In two recent reviews in 1971 by Adams and Fetterhoff, and 1972 by Khunda there appear to have been a further 49 cases added to the literature. Nissen in his review divided the twin entanglements into four categories:

1. Collision. The contact of any fetal parts of one twin with those of its co-twin preventing engagement of either.
2. Impaction. The impaction of any fetal parts of one twin into the surface of its co-twin permitting partial engagement of both simultaneously.
3. Compaction. The simultaneous full engagement of the leading fetal poles of both twins filling the two pelvic cavities and preventing further descent or disengagement of either.

4. Interlocking. The intimate adhesion of the inferior surface of a twin's chin with that of its co-twin above or below the pelvic inlet.

   The aetiology of locking has been variously ascribed to small fetuses, a large pelvis, deficiency of amniotic fluid, premature rupture of the membranes, the use of oxytocics and hypertonicity of the uterus. Primiparity has also been suggested by Lawrence in 1949 as a predisposing factor because he found that in a review of 28 cases there were 23 primigravidas. This finding was

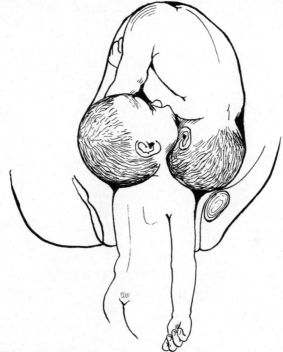

Figure 11.2. Chin-to-chin locking in twins.

confirmed by Khunda (1972) in his further series of locked twins in which he found that primiparas were almost twice as common as multigravidas. It has been suggested that the high tone of the lower uterine segment in the primigravid patient might predispose to the impaction or locking.

   The diagnosis cannot be predicted before the onset of labour and is not usually detected until part of the first baby has been born. The condition might be suspected if the labour is prolonged or is not pursuing a normal course.

PRESENTATION

In the series of 37 cases reported by Khunda (1972) the following presentations were found: breech/vertex, 31; vertex/vertex, 4; vertex/breech, 1;

shoulder/shoulder, 1. Breech/vertex is then by far the most common presentation. The commonest way for twins to present is vertex/vertex, but it is obvious that breech/vertex presentation is by far the most common for locking.

UTERINE ABNORMALITY

Although this is uncommon it has been twice reported as a cause of locked twins (Parmar and Mulgund, 1968; Theron, 1969).

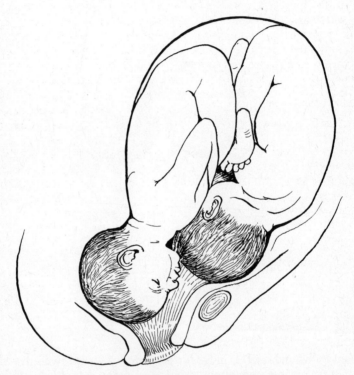

Figure 11.3. Collision of two heads causing a form of locked twins.

MANAGEMENT OF INTERLOCKED TWINS

There is no standardised technique for the delivery of interlocked twins as no one has had a sufficiently large personal series of this rare complication to develop a standard plan of management. If the condition is suspected in labour then an x-ray should be taken and if the condition is confirmed Caesarean section should be carried out. Unfortunately, the diagnosis is not usually made until the first twin is partially born. The condition may not be recognised until fairly strenuous efforts have been made to deliver the first baby by traction, but if at all possible a strong traction on the first baby should be avoided. When the diagnosis has been made a careful assessment is made to determine the degree of locking and whether it will be possible to disengage the heads. It is probably preferable to do this under a general anaesthesia and to deepen the anaesthesia so that disengagement of the heads can be carried out. This, however, is unlikely to be possible because all of the liquor will have drained away. In that case the Kimball and Rand (1950) procedure should be carried out. After checking that there is pulsation in the cord of the first baby the procedure is carried out as follows: forceps are applied to the head of the second twin and traction and hyperextension are applied to the first twin. The head of the second twin is delivered by flexion. There is danger in this manoeuvre to the maternal tissues. If the first twin is dead then decapitation is carried out and the second twin is born as expeditiously as possible. Caesarean section is not of value where there is chin to chin interlocking and the first baby is partially born, but in some cases it may be possible to deliver both twins through a classical Caesarean section incision. The Kimball–Rand manoeuvre is only helpful when the babies are small. If the babies are large there is too much danger of causing damage to the maternal tissues.

Locking of triplets has also been reported by Swann (1957). Locking occurred between the first and second infants. It was possible in this case to push up the head of the second infant under a general anaesthesia and deliver the first baby.

PERINATAL MORTALITY IN LOCKED TWINS

In Khunda's 1972 series of the 74 babies, 21 died at delivery giving a fetal mortality of 31 per cent. In Nissen's series of 70 cases, there were 59 perinatal deaths. The first baby born is more likely to die than the second when the babies are interlocked.

THIRD STAGE

It is unusual for the first placenta in a dichorionic twin pregnancy to be delivered before the second baby, but it does not seem to cause any harm to the second twin. If it is quite certain that there are only two babies present then ergometrine or syntometrine or speeding up of the syntocinon infusion should be carried out after the delivery of the second twin and the placenta or placentas delivered with controlled cord traction.

Although it used to be thought that postpartum haemorrhage was more common in multiple pregnancies because of overdistension and inertia of the uterus this is now known not to be so (Wood and Pinkerton, 1966), and haemorrhage is no more common than after a singleton delivery provided that oxytocics are given and controlled cord traction is employed.

DELIVERY OF TRIPLETS AND HIGHER MULTIPLES

Provided that there are no complications or contraindications it is usual to deliver triplets vaginally, but when there are four or more babies recourse to Caesarean section is more readily made unless the labour starts spontaneously pre-term, i.e., before 37 weeks. It is essential that in the delivery of multiple births there is an adequate staff available, both of obstetricians and paediatricians. There should be one paediatrician for each baby and resuscitation equipment for each should also be available (Fullerton et al, 1965; McFee et al, 1974). The former authors delivered by Caesarean section and the latter authors delivered both sets of quadruplets vaginally, one set at 30 and the other at 35 weeks. In the two cases of McFee and his co-workers no attempt was made to stop the premature labour either with a β-adrenergic stimulator or with a cervical suture. The famous Dionne quintuplets were delivered spontaneously at home and it is remarkable how they survived (Da Foe, 1934).

It seems reasonable to argue that in higher multiple births Caesarean section should be more readily made recourse to because each succeeding baby in the multiple pregnancy is probably at higher risk judging from the greater risk of the second baby in a twin pregnancy compared to the first.

CHAPTER 12

Malformations and Other Abnormalities in Twins

I. MACGILLIVRAY

The study of malformations in twins is of interest and importance from two points of view. Firstly, it may be possible to distinguish genetic from intra-uterine factors in the causation of malformation depending on whether the malformation occurred in only one or in both twins, in monozygotic or dizygotic pregnancies. Twins share a similar intrauterine environment but may have either identical heredity as is the case with monozygotic twins, or dissimilar heredity as is the case of the dizygotic twins. Secondly, the possibility of a more frequent occurrence of malformation in twins compared to singletons is of interest. It is known that most congenital malformations increase in incidence with increasing age of the mother. This is comparable to the increasing incidence of twins with age and possibly accounts for some of the higher incidence of malformations in twin pregnancies than in singletons. Parity, however, does not have the same effect as malformations are commoner in primigravidae.

The majority of reports are agreed that there is an increased incidence of malformations in twins with the notable exception of McKeown and Record (1960) who found that in a series of 1550 twins there were 21 malformed which is not significantly above the number expected if malformations were unrelated to plurality. Hendricks (1966) found that amongst 758 twins the anomaly rate was 10.6 per cent compared with 3.3 per cent for all births but the anomalies were not clearly defined.

From a study of the records of 21 000 pairs of twins, Gittlesohn and Milham (1964) found a higher incidence of malformations among like-sexed pair twins than among unlike-sexed twins, but they did not give comparable data for single births. A higher incidence of malformations was noted in a small series of twins among monozygotic than among dizygotic twins by Fogel, Nitowsky and Greenwold (1965). In an analysis of consecutive births from

24 centres throughout the world, Stevenson et al (1966) reported a higher rate of congenital malformations among twins than singletons which was accounted for by individuals from like-sexed pairs. A higher incidence of malformations in twins than in singletons has also been reported by Guttmacher and Kohl (1958) and Pedlow (1961).

As pointed out by Hay and Wehrung (1970), who have reported the largest series so far of about 4000 twins, one of the greatest limitations encountered in studying congenital malformations in twins is the difficulty of obtaining a large enough series for reliable results. For example, in the U.S.A. the incidence of cleft lip and/or palate, which is one of the most common malformations, is reported as one in every 800 babies born. As about one in every 50 babies born alive is a twin, it would be necessary to observe about 40 000 live births in order to detect one with a cleft palate. The alternative method is to study a series of twins which have been collected without reference to the total births. This is liable to introduce errors as it is likely that such a series will contain an over-representation of concordant twins and an under-representation of cases where a co-twin has died. Concordance means that both twins are affected. Carter (1965) in his review of the literature pointed out that few large-scale studies of co-twins of index patients with common congenital malformations have been carried out.

Two such studies based on all cases in a population have been reported by Idelberger for talipes equinovarus (1939) and congenital dislocation of the hip (1951). The type of twinning was determined by physical resemblance and not by blood group. There were 29 monozygotic pairs with congenital dislocation of the hip of whom 10, all females, were both affected. If both were index patients in each of the concordant pairs the proportion of co-twins of index patients affected would be 20 in 39, or 51.3 per cent. If only one in each pair was an index patient the proportion would be 34.5 per cent. In contrast none of 52 like-sexed dizygotic twins were concordant, whilst three of 57 unlike-sexed twins were concordant. The overall number of affected dizygotic twins of index patients was six in 112, i.e. 5.4 per cent since all affected were index patients. From this series it appears that genetic factors play a major role in the causation of congenital dislocation of the hip but environmental factors are also important. Similarly, Idelberger found that the genetic factors played a major part in the causation of talipes equinovarus. There were 35 monozygotic pairs of whom eight (22.9 per cent) were concordant. In five pairs both were index patients giving a concordance of 32.5 per cent. In contrast only three of 133 dizygotic pairs were concordant and in one pair both were index patients giving a concordance of three per cent.

The concordance rates for cleft lip and cleft palate reported by Metrakos, Metrakos and Baxter (1958) and Douglas (1958) were remarkably similar being 31 per cent and 30 per cent for monozygotic twins and six per cent and five per cent for dizygotic twins respectively. In Hay and Wehrung's large 1970 series, the estimated concordance rates for cleft lip with or without cleft palate were 17.6 per cent monozygotic and 2.4 per cent dizygotic, and for cleft palate alone 40 per cent monozygotic and 4.8 per cent dizygotic.

In the series of Hay and Wehrung (1970) the incidence of the majority of selected malformations was increased in like-sexed twins but not in unlike-sexed twins (Table 12.1), but cleft lip and palate and polydactyly did not show any differences. Congenital heart disease was much more frequent in like-sexed twins than in the other two groups. This is similar to McKeown and Record's (1960) finding that there was a higher proportion of twins with cardiac malformations but the difference was not significant. The proportion of like-sexed twins was also considerably in excess of that expected. In the central nervous system malformations (Table 12.1) both anencephaly and hydro-

Table 12.1. *Incidence of congenital malformations per 100 000 live births.*

	Single deliveries	Unlike-sexed twin deliveries	Like-sexed twin deliveries
Cleft lip and palate	47.5	39.9	41.6
Anencephaly	23.2	21.5	44.6
Spina bifida	62.5	46.0	61.7
Hydrocephaly	30.2	30.7	44.6
Heart disease	58.9	49.1	81.0
Polydactyly	89.3	87.4	93.7
Down's syndrome	43.5	35.3	24.5

Adapted from Hay, S. L., Wehrung, D. A. (1970).

cephaly were more common in the like-sexed group than in the other two groups and spina bifida was less common in unlike-sexed twins than in the other two groups. Males in the like-sexed pairs tended to be more affected by anencephaly and spina bifida than males in unlike-sexed pairs or in single births. McKeown and Record (1960) also found a high incidence of twins among hydrocephalics relative to the population of total births, but they did not find any increase in the incidence of anencephaly or spina bifida.

Carter also concluded from a review of the available literature that only a minority of monozygotic co-twins of index patients with anencephaly and spina bifida cystica are also affected and that there is no clear indication that this proportion is any higher than that of dizygotic twins also affected. On the other hand, Scott and Paterson (1966) reported a very interesting case of monozygotic anencephalic triplets. The placenta was triamniotic and mono-chorial, the fetal blood groups were identical and the circulations were linked.

Gellman (1959) and Larson and Banner (1966) have reported monoamniotic twins discordant for hydrocephalus but there were no reports of such twins concordant for hydrocephalus until Larson, Wilson and Titus (1969) reported a case of monoamniotic twin pregnancy in which both twins had hydro-cephalus and meningomyelocele.

McKeown and Record (1960) found that in their series of 1550 twins there were 463 like-sexed pairs with 26 malformed twins, and 311 unlike-sexed pairs with 15 malformed. Among the like-sexed pairs there were two examples of partial concordance and among unlike-sexed pairs there was one of partial concordance and one of possible concordance (each twin had cardiac malformations of unspecified nature).

The concordance rates for malformations in Hay and Wehrung's series where the zygosity was determined by Weinberg's formula were within the range expected on the basis of previous studies of twins with known zygosity, but there was an excess occurrence of monozygotic twins with central nervous system malformations (112 out of 222 total pairs, or 50.5 per cent), and congenital heart defects (69 out of 129, or 53.5 per cent). These rates imply a stronger genetic component in clefts and polydactyly than in central nervous system malformations and congenital heart disease. They also found that twins from unlike-sexed pairs had fewer additional malformations associated with congenital heart disease, polydactyly, and Down's syndrome, than did twins from like-sexed pairs or singletons. With these exceptions the proportion of index cases having at least one additional malformation was strikingly similar for twins of both sex types and singletons.

Twin studies indicate that all the common malformations such as hare lip, with or without cleft palate, talipes equinovarus, polydactyly, cardiac malformations and congenital dislocation of the hip must be, in part, environmentally determined but also give a strong indication, except perhaps in the case of anencephalus, spina bifida and hydrocephalus, that genetic factors are also important. Hay and Wehrung (1970) suggest that the relatively high incidence associated with low concordance of anencephaly, hydrocephaly and cardiac malformations in like-sexed twins indicates that placental anastomosis may play an important role in the occurrence of these malformations.

For most malformations for which the evidence is available the degree of concordance appears to be little if any higher in monozygotic than in dizygotic twins.

MONGOLISM IN TWINS

In mongolism or Down's syndrome there is a third chromosome instead of the usual pair, most commonly of chromosome 21 (trisomy [21]). This usually occurs by non-disjunction but can also occur by translocation to other chromosomes.

Mongolism is no more common in twins than in singleton children, but as pointed out by Bulmer (1970) monozygotic twins must be concordant for mongolism except in the rare event of the abnormality occurring after fertilisation. Dizygotic twins, on the other hand, are rarely concordant for mongolism because they require two separate chromosomal abnormalities.

MacDonald reviewed the literature to 1964 to try to determine a more accurate estimate than previously of the true ratio of concordant to discordant pairs, and received reports on 71 pairs in which the diagnosis of mongolism was confirmed from obstetricians in Britain. The 67 twin pairs were studied in which a diagnosis of mongolism in one or both infants was made. Two pairs of unlike-sex were concordant for mongolism whereas, allowing for maternal age, 0.14 pairs would have been expected. This suggests that some women have a tendency over and above that due to maternal age to produce affected children. There were five pairs of twins of like-sex concordant for mongolism. Allowing for the known relationship between the maternal age and twinning 10.5 monozygotic pairs would have been expected. Assuming that monozygotic twins are almost always concordant for mongolism there were about half as many pairs as expected. Since in the 60 discordant pairs there was an equal number of pairs of like and unlike-sex (30 of each) there was nothing to suggest the presence of monozygotic discordant pairs. Keay (1958) found one concordant pair in 11 pairs of unlike-sex, a similar proportion to that found in MacDonald's study. However, in general, it can no longer be assumed that monozygotic twins are always concordant for mongolism as three accurately diagnosed monozygotic discordant pairs have so far been reported (Scott and Ferguson-Smith, 1973). Hay and Wehrung (1970) found that Down's syndrome was less common in both types of twins than in single births, but probably this was due to fetal deaths being excluded from their series. They found a deficiency of monozygotic twins with Down's syndrome (five out of 51, 9.8 per cent) which they suggested implied a high genetic component in this condition.

The very high concordance rate in Down's syndrome among like-sexed twins along with a relatively low incidence suggests that there is an early loss of affected monozygotic embryos due to a combination of the effects of zygote cleavage and chromosomal imbalance.

SEXUAL ANOMALIES IN TWINS

Halbert and Christakos (1970) reported a case of uterus didelphys in one of twins presumed to be monozygotic on the basis of blood group studies. Her sister had normal uterine development. De George (1970) in a study of 329 mothers of twins found that seven mothers of twins had affected members of twin pairs in that the boys had hypospadias and the girls had an enlarged clitoris, whereas none of the boys or girls of the mothers of singletons were affected. There were members in five like-sexed male pairs with hypospadias, two pairs concordant and three discordant, and one female member each of a like-sexed and unlike-sexed pair had an enlarged clitoris. The zygosity of the like-sexed pair was not determined. A case of double aploidy has been reported in a pair of monozygotic twins. They had both mongolism and Klinefelter's syndrome.

CONJOINED TWINS

If there is imperfect division of the embryo after the formation of two embryonic areas then conjoined twins or double monsters occur. The possibilities of survival of conjoined twins depends on such factors as the degree of separation, the site of union, the sharing of vital organs, and the presence or absence of other defects. Modern surgical techniques have enabled the successful separation of twins who have had quite an extensive fusion and it is therefore important that the baby should be born in the best condition possible. Unfortunately, the diagnosis is liable to be missed before birth because of the extreme rarity of the condition and the diagnosis is not considered.

In a series reported in 1971 by Tan et al from Singapore (Tan et al, 1971a) there was an incidence of one in 57 975 deliveries and one in 546 in twin deliveries. Compton, also in 1971, reported an incidence of one in 50 000 and estimated an incidence of one in 900 twin gestations. Mudaliar (1930) reported an incidence of four in 25 000 deliveries in India, Mortimer and Kirschbaum (1942) three in 85 000 and Scammon (1925) two in 100 000. The most famous of conjoined twins were the Siamese twins Chang and Eng Bunker who appeared in Barnum's circus in America. As there is no hereditary factor in monozygotic twinning it is not surprising that in more than

Dicephalus   Syncephalus

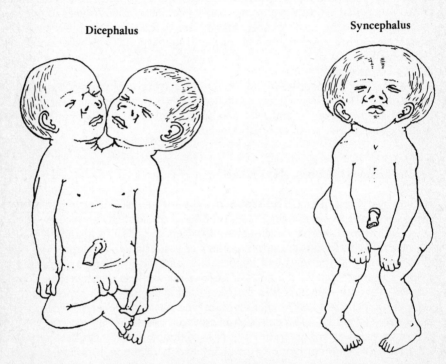

Figure 12.1. Two types of double monsters: (a) dicephalus with one trunk and two heads; (b) syncephalus with a shared trunk and conjoined heads.

1000 of their descendants there has only recently been one reported incidence of twin pregnancy (Aird, 1959).

Any part of the bodies may be joined but the common types as reported by Tartuffi quoted by Tan et al (1971a) in a series of 117 cases were 86 of thoracopagus, 32 pyopagus, 7 ischiopagus and 2 craniopagus. In some cases there is incomplete duplication so that organs are shared. For example, there may be only one heart or one liver. The whole trunk may be shared and these are really cases of double monsters as in dicephalus with one trunk and two heads and syncephalus with a shared trunk and conjoined heads (Figure 12.1). Thoracopagus twins are joined in thee pigastric and thoracic regions (Figure 12.2), pyopagus at the pelvis, ischiopagus laterally at the pelvis and craniopagus by the head.

The survival of these twins is dependent on the degree of abnormality. When the heads are joined as in craniopagus the survival is dependent on highly skilled operative procedures to effect separation. Thoracopagus presents a good chance of survival and normal development, provided that vital organs are not shared.

Thoracopagus

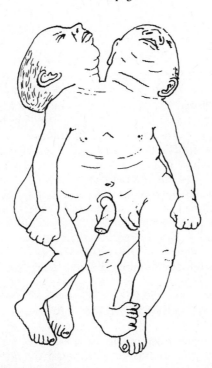

Figure 12.2. Thoracopagus twins.

The diagnosis is rarely made antepartum (Rudolph, Michaels and Nichols, 1967). It is dependent on a twin pregnancy being suspected or if hydramnios is present and further investigation with x-rays reveals that the twins are conjoined. Rudolph et al pointed out that there was a greater incidence of hydramnios with conjoined twins (76 per cent) compared to normal twins (10 per cent). Radiologically the diagnosis may be made (i) if the twins face one another, (ii) the fetal heads are at the same level and plane, (iii) the thoracic cages of the fetuses are together or in proximity, (iv) the presence of extreme dorsiflexion of the cervical spines, and (v) the relative position of the fetuses does not change with movement, manipulation, or after repeat films at a later time. These criteria do not apply to vertex presentations. Sonar scanning could be of help, but so far no report has been made of any scan of conjoined twins.

The diagnosis is often not made until labour is advanced. If there is only soft tissue union dystocia does not arise but if there is dystocia with a twin pregnancy in the presence of active labour, then the possibility of conjoined twins, fetal interlocking, or fetal abnormalities must be considered.

If the diagnosis is made when the twins are of a reasonable size, delivery by elective Caesarean section should be aimed at. A difficult destructive operation is more likely to cause damage to the mother and should preferably be avoided.

FETUS PAPYRACEUS

When one twin dies at a fairly late stage in development from such conditions as transfusion syndrome, cord compression or haemolytic disease, it shrinks and becomes compressed by the living twin into the chorion laeve of the placenta. This is known as a fetus papyraceus or compressus and it may be overlooked especially if it is small. This condition can also occur in higher multiples and Potter (1961) has reported a case in which one monochorionic triplet went to term while the other two died from entangled cords in a mono-amniotic sac and became papyraceus fetuses.

Kindred reviewed the literature in 1944 and found that 66 per cent of 141 cases of fetus papyraceus twins with adequate information were dichorionic and two per cent were monoamniotic. The diagnosis of fetus papyraceus is not commonly made until it is delivered, usually along with the placenta of the surviving twin. Benirschke and Driscoll (1967) describe the various appearances of papyraceus fetuses found by different authors.

ACARDIAC AND ACEPHALIC MONSTERS

Acardiac monsters occur only in monozygotic, monochorionic twin pregnancies in which the circulations are linked and the normal fetus supports the acardiac twin. According to Benirschke and Driscoll (1967) the occurrence of acardiac twins has always occurred in one of what are judged to be single ovum twins with monochorial placenta. Occasionally, it has been seen in one of triplets or even quintuplets, at least one of them being monochorial with the acardiac. An umbilical cord is typically present in the acardiac and in most cases it contains but one artery and one vein. In five cases of amorphous acardiac twins the sex chromatin was found to be identical with that of the associated normal twin. In another acardiac fetus who weighed much in excess of the normal partner skin tissue cultures were used for chromosome preparations. The normal twin was male and the karyotypes from the monster were normal male. These cases, as those in which gonads have been found, support the single ovum derivation of acardiacs by their universally identical sex. They support also the notion that vascular events are the cause of the anomaly. The frequency of acardiac twins is difficult to assess and has been estimated at one in 34 600 deliveries (one per cent of monozygous twins) by Gillim and Hendricks (1953). The acardius acephalus is the most common possibly because of the proximity of the lower portion of the body to the entering blood and the amorphi the rarest. Many exercises in classification of these malformations have been carried out, but these are probably somewhat meaningless as their pathogenesis is probably similar (Benirschke and Kim, 1973).

Two main theories (Keith, Cestaro and Elias, 1967; Wilson, 1972) are held about the origin of acardia and related monsters: one states (Alderman, 1973; Severn and Holyoke, 1973) that the defect is a primary one, in other words the heart was never present, and the other view, favoured by Schatz and discussed by Benirschke and Driscoll (1967), holds that there was a heart but that this subsequently atrophies as a result of imbalance in the placental vascular communications. Chromosomal anomalies have been found in acardiac monsters (Scott and Ferguson-Smith, 1973), but they are not invariably associated with the anomaly (Severn and Holyoke, 1973) and it seems likely that they might be a secondary event (Turpin, Bocquet and Grasset, 1967). Acardia has been described in cattle (placental vascular communications are usually present in such twins) and recently chromosome studies were carried out in such a case, the twins being found to be of unlike-sex and therefore DZ (Dunn, Lein and Kenney, 1967). Thus 'unequal splitting' of a single zygote which has been one of the hypotheses put forward for their origin, cannot now be held to be responsible and it seems more likely that there is atrophy of the heart as a result of some form of malfunction in the common placental circulation (Benirschke, 1972a; Benirschke and Kim, 1973).

CHIMERISM

A chimera was a mythological fire-spouting monster with a lion's head, a goat's body, and a snake's tail, but in medicine the term chimera is applied to dizygotic twins whose blood was originally of different groups but in whom there has been an interchange of blast cells in utero so that their bloods are of mixed groups. The chances of vascular communication in fused dichorial placentas have been estimated at between one in 100 and one in 1000 by Strong and Corney (1967). When this occurs it probably gives rise to blood chimerism in human twins. In this condition red blood cells of two distinct blood groups are found in each of the twins.

In cattle, and to a lesser extent in sheep, goats and pigs, the female member of unlike-sexed twins is usually sterile and known as a freemartin, but this situation is unknown in man and the marmoset monkey. The freemartin effect was originally thought to be produced by male hormone passing across the anastomosis, but this explanation is now thought to be untenable as androgens given to pregnant cows do not interfere with normal ovarian development (Jost, 1970, 1974). It seems more likely that some factor, as yet unidentified, may cross from the male thus inducing the female gonad to produce male-type hormones (Short, 1970). An alternative explanation is that, in addition to other cells, primordial germ cells might be exchanged along the vascular freeway and subsequently be responsible for the sex anomaly, but this hypothesis has also yet to be proven (Short, 1970; Bishop, 1972). Thus no solution is at present to hand for this riddle of apparent intra-uterine male domination. In the field of immunology the effect is a profound one, for such twins, even though DZ, are immunologically tolerant of each other to the extent that each will accept skin grafts from the co-twin, though not necessarily indefinitely (for discussion see Benirschke, 1970).

Although placental anastomosis and chimerism have been demonstrated in the marmoset, the freemartin effect is not seen (Benirschke, 1970) and it is observed rarely, if at all, in similar circumstances in the mare (Vandeplassche, Podliachouk and Beaud, 1970). An important factor in the variability of manifestations between species might be differences in the relative develop-mental timing of the placental anastomoses and sexual differentiation (Benir-schke, 1970; Jeffcott and Whitwell, 1973).

Man also escapes the freemartin effect apparently. A number of human blood chimeras have now been described (Race and Sanger, 1975); these have usually been detected when mixed populations of cells were noticed, often at blood transfusion centres. The person concerned in some cases was unaware that he or she was a twin, the co-twin having died at or shortly after birth. Relatively few such human chimeras have been found, but the females have usually been fertile and hence there must be some fundamental difference here between a girl and a heifer which has so far eluded (reproductive bio-logical) discovery.

HYDATIDIFORM MOLE IN TWIN PREGNANCY

According to Chamberlain (1963) twin gestation is statistically more common in association with hydatidiform mole than without this association. In some cases one placenta may be transformed into a hydatidiform mole with disappearance of the fetus, or if changes occur at later stages of pregnancy the affected placenta may show only partial molar degeneration with con-tinuing fetal growth. Absence of one umbilical artery occurs frequently perhaps as often as once in one hundred deliveries. In abortion it occurs in 2.4 to 2.7 per cent. It is seen more frequently still in twins and it may occur in one of monozygous twins or in both, and is most frequently the case in acardiacs. It may also be present in both of dizygous twins.

ABORTION IN TWIN PREGNANCY

It is difficult to determine the frequency of twinning in spontaneous abortions because the aborted material is often disrupted particularly in the very early gestations. Javert (1957) quotes frequencies ranging from six per cent to 20 per cent, but in his own series there were only 24 cases in 2000 abortions (1.2 per cent) and Benirschke and Driscoll (1967) found only 0.3 per cent in their 1870 abortions. It is striking, however, that only one was dichorial and heterosexual but there were four diamniotic monochorionic and two monoamniotic twins. One of the latter showed the classical entangling of cords considered by Quigley (1935) to be responsible for the abortion of 24 of 109 monoamniotic twins. Guttmacher (1937) found one twin abortion amongst 37.1 abortions as compared to one in 86.5 viable births, but unfortunately they were not divided on the basis of the number of membranes. There is then possibly a greater loss of monozygous compared to dizygous twins in the early embryonic period than in viable twins.

Potter (1963) says "the proportionate number of twin pregnancies that terminate in abortion is not greatly in excess of those terminating after the twentieth to twenty-second week". It seems likely therefore that twin pregnancies are not more common amongst abortions but the twins that are found are usually monochorionic.

CHAPTER 13

Neonatal Care

V. FARR

Apart from the twin-transfusion syndrome and operative separation of conjoined twins, multiple births have no specific neonatal problems and their postnatal management depends mainly on birthweight, gestational age and the type of delivery. As a group they are more likely to be pre-term, small-for-dates and have a complicated delivery, so their neonatal care should be geared to these problems. The principal determining factors in the survival of these small infants are the quality of nursing care, the standard of medical attention and the availability of specialised monitoring and therapeutic facilities (Leading Article, *British Medical Journal*, 1970).

GENERAL CONSIDERATIONS

The pre-term infant is anatomically and physiologically immature and this is especially apparent in the respiratory system, where sustained respiration is often delayed at birth, and once started is usually laboured. Poor oxygenation may result from pulmonary atelectasis, hyaline membrane or a combination of these. Apnoeic attacks due to poor cerebral function may be aggravated by intra-ventricular haemorrhage, especially if this is also associated with birth asphyxia. Temperature control may be poor, not only because of an incompetent autonomic nervous system, but because the sweat glands are immature (Green and Behrendt, 1973). An inadequately developed gastro-intestinal system means feeding problems which may add to the iron and vitamin deficiencies of the later neonatal period. Iron storage in the liver and kidneys doubles in the last weeks of gestation and the smaller and further from term the baby, the lower the iron reserves (Chang, 1973). Prolonged and sometimes severe jaundice may result from hepatic immaturity and if the reticuloendothelial system is below par this increases the risk of anaemia as well as adding to the susceptibility to infection (Schaffer, 1963; Robinson, 1971a).

176

The problems of the low birthweight baby who is also small-for-dates are somewhat different to those of the pre-term infant. Birth asphyxia, hypoglycaemia, intrapulmonary haemorrhage and polycythaemia are his major difficulties (Robinson, 1971b). Asphyxia and malformation are three times as common as in the general population and hypoglycaemia is six times more frequent. Polycythaemia is twice as common as one might expect and more than half of those who have polycythaemia are severely asphyxiated at birth (Lugo and Cassady, 1971). About ten per cent of babies whose birthweight is below the tenth percentile for gestation have some congenital abnormality (Ounsted and Ounsted, 1973).

Difficult or operative delivery may result in birth trauma such as intracranial haemorrhage, fractures, or peripheral nerve palsies and an increased risk of birth asphyxia.

It is obvious that with all these potential difficulties these babies must be born in units where specialised paediatric care is available immediately, if they are to have the best chance of living a normal healthy life. As well as this, transfer to a special care unit after delivery not only involves a waste of precious time but transportation may be an extra hazard which they can ill afford. Furthermore, it means that the mother is separated from her babies (perhaps by a great distance) at a time when she is emotionally less able to cope with additional problems.

Situations which may involve the obstetrician, such as resuscitation, and conditions specific to multiple births will be dealt with in detail, but other neonatal problems will be looked at with a view to helping the obstetrician answer questions which might be put to him by the parents before or after the babies are born. The management described in this chapter is based on the routine care in the labour ward and the special care nursery of the Aberdeen Maternity Hospital. Further suggested reading for those interested will be found in Brown and Valman (1971).

RESUSCITATION

Babies resulting from multiple pregnancies are not only liable to be delivered before term, but malpresentation and operative delivery are common, so that those in attendance should anticipate trouble long before it occurs, and they should ensure that there are enough trained personnel and equipment to cope with the resuscitation of each baby. The firstborn usually presents by the vertex (Butler and Alberman, 1969), and resuscitation problems are less likely, but any delay in delivering the second (and subsequent) baby may cause cerebral depression, and sustained respiration may not be initiated for several minutes, if at all, without adequate help. At least one attendant should be able to pass an endotracheal tube, be capable of dealing with a severely asphyxiated baby and have sufficient neonatal experience to assess the need for further medical or surgical care.

The days of vigorous resuscitation by immersing the baby in water of varying (and sometimes extreme) temperature, or by the use of strong stimulants are past, but there is still no universal agreement on how birth asphyxia should be treated. The nasal airway should be cleared by gentle suction. Repeated over-enthusiastic suction, especially around the area of the larynx, leads to cardiorespiratory depression, and does not act as a stimulus to respiration. If respiration is not established immediately, slapping the soles of the feet may give the necessary impetus. Suspending the baby by the feet, or maintaining him in an exaggerated head-down position are not recommended, as the pressure of the abdominal viscera reduces diaphragmatic movement. If the infant gasps occasionally, oxygen should be given by funnel, not by a mask clamped down on the face. If apnoea persists and the heart rate is less than 100 per minute, oxygen should be given by endotracheal tube. If this cannot be done expertly, mouth-to-face resuscitation is probably more beneficial and less traumatic than incompetent intubation. Pressure chambers are still in use in some units but they have little or no place where there is a paediatrician within easy reach of the delivery room. Intravenous Lorfan (levallorphan) may be needed if the mother was sedated within an hour or two of delivery and it is felt that the babies' respiratory depression is due to this, but it is probably better to give Lorfan to the mother before they are born. Intravenous sodium bicarbonate may be of help when intrauterine hypoxia has been prolonged, but it should be used with care, since it can only be given on an empirical basis, as there is no time to await biochemical results.

Most asphyxiated neonates do well once respiration is established and it is only those who have suffered marked cerebral anoxia who have residual problems in the neonatal period. Continuing respiratory difficulty may be due to many causes, not necessarily pulmonary, and those who do not recover fully within an hour of birth should be admitted to a specialised unit for further investigation. Infants with evidence of brain damage may not recover within the first few days and in these cases it is often difficult to determine which came first, the cerebral impairment or the asphyxia, and this may be one reason why there are conflicting views on the long-term effects of birth asphyxia. It may be that the underlying cause of the asphyxia is of more prognostic significance than its severity, but on principle it is better that any degree of asphyxia should last for as short a time as possible, especially in small and pre-term babies, who are less well equipped to cope with a reduced oxygen supply (Schaffer, 1963).

Once the child has recovered from the delivery the nursing care outlined by Smellie over two hundred years ago still holds true: ". . . the principal aim at this point is to keep the child's head and body neither too tight nor too slovenly, too hot nor too cold; that it may be warm, though not overheated, and easy, though not too loose; that respiration may be full and large . . ." (Smellie, 1752).

As soon as the babies' general condition is satisfactory, they should be examined for birth injury and malformation, not only to instigate investigations and treatment where these are indicated, but in the majority of cases to reassure the mother that all is well.

TWIN-TRANSFUSION SYNDROME

This problem arises when transfusion occurs in utero between identical twins, probably over a long period (see also Chapters 3 and 10). The babies show disparities in weight, skin colour and haemoglobin levels, the plethoric recipient often being in a worse clinical condition than the smaller, anaemic donor. The plethoric twin has a high cord haemoglobin and a high haematocrit, and often exhibits peripheral cyanosis even when only mildly hypoxic. If the polycythaemia is marked there may be cerebral irritation and convulsions, with the added risk of cerebral thrombosis. Apnoeic attacks, respiratory difficulties, hyperbilirubinaemia, hypoglycaemia and thrombocytopenia are other possible complications (Shorland, 1971; Cross, Hathaway and McGaughey, 1973). The donor twin may be grossly anaemic and if small-for-dates may also become hypoglycaemic. Birth asphyxia, heart failure, respiratory failure, cardiac arrest, hypothermia and generalised convulsions all occurred in the case reported by Shorland (1971) and this baby was extremely ill for several days.

All like-sex twins with marked birthweight differences should have venous (not capillary) blood tested for haemoglobin and haematocrit levels, in both babies. In many cases no treatment will be necessary, but if their general condition is poor, or the recipient's haematocrit is above 70 per cent, partial exchange transfusion may be necessary, using plasma for the recipient and packed cells for the donor, to correct the cardiovascular and red cell imbalance (Davies et al, 1972).

A high rise in blood viscosity increases the risk of vascular thrombosis and heart failure, and prophylactic treatment should be considered in all cases. Venesection is slow and may lead to hypovolaemia before the haematocrit level is reduced. Repeated replacement transfusions of 40 ml of plasma or albumin for every 50 ml blood removed, taking 10 ml aliquots, to reduce the haematocrit to below 70 per cent, have been advocated by Sacks (1959) but if the serum bilirubin rises, a standard exchange transfusion, with whole blood, will not only reduce the bilirubin level but will also lower the haematocrit. The anaemia in the donor twin is best treated by exchange transfusion with packed cells, and repeated partial transfusions may be necessary if the general condition is very poor (Shorland, 1971).

Heart failure may present with tachypnoea, intercostal indrawing and failure to feed. Cardiac murmurs, gallop rhythm, moist sounds on auscultation and an abnormal cardiac outline on x-ray differentiate it from hyaline membrane disease. Treatment consists of digitalisation, diuretics, oxygen and sedation if the baby if very restless. The suggested regimen for digitalisation is 0.04 mg per kg of oral Lanoxin initially, then 0.02 mg per kg six-hourly for two or three doses, and then daily thereafter. The equivalent intramuscular dose is 0.015 mg per kg. If a diuretic is needed, frusemide (Lasix) 2 mg per kg can be given every one to two days. The baby is usually more comfortable if he is nursed propped up, and a warm environment prevents unnecessary oxygen utilisation and counteracts hypothermia.

Intravenous sodium bicarbonate may be required to correct respiratory acidosis. This should be given into a peripheral rather than the umbilical vein, because of the complications which may arise (such as thrombosis and embolism; Messer et al, 1972) when using the latter. The dosage must be monitored by Pao_2 estimations, and in severe cases, with recurrent apnoeic attacks and a high Pco_2, mechanical ventilation may be required.

High calorie feeds (reconstituted with 10 per cent Caloreen instead of water) or breast milk, are preferable to intravenous therapy in the prevention of hypoglycaemia, the latter being reserved for those with symptoms, or when oral feeding is not possible. Once intravenous therapy has been started care must be taken when changing over to oral feeding as reactive hypoglycaemia is common at this time (Robinson, 1971b).

CONJOINED TWINS

The majority of conjoined twins (75 per cent) are thoracopagus and omphalopagus, and the least common type is craniopagus (two per cent). The first recorded separation of conjoined twins was in 1689, and until the 20th century these early cases were omphalopagus twins. The first thoracopagus separation was in 1900. In more recent times, 11 omphalopagus and xiphopagus pairs have been operated upon, their ages varying from a few hours to 13 years old. All but three infants survived. Seven attempts at separating thoracopagus twins with separate hearts have been recorded, the operations being done at one day to three months of age. Only six babies survived separation. Of three cases of thoracopagus with conjoined hearts none survived the operation (Nichols, Blattner and Rudolph, 1967).

Whether or not separation is possible depends on many factors, and where there are shared organs, moral and ethical problems must be considered if separation means sacrificing one twin to save the other. Co-existing malformations are common, and if they are both severe and discordant they are bound to affect the decision regarding separation for the benefit of one twin. If separation is feasible, preparations for and the timing of the operation are important in relation to survival.

Despite the large number of case reports in the literature, few contain details which are helpful in assessing the chances of successful separation in an individual case. Nichols, Blattner and Rudolph (1967) in a comprehensive review of thoracopagus twins gave details of investigation, management and prognosis, and Simpson (1969) also gave a full account of the management of one case from birth until after operation.

The degree of cardiovascular conjunction must be determined before surgery is contemplated, as 75 per cent of thoracopagus twins have conjoined hearts. If separate ventricular contractions can be detected clinically the prognosis for separation is good. Simultaneous palpation of independent femoral pulses in each twin is a reliable indication of independent ventricles (Nichols, Blattner and Rudolph, 1967; Simpson, 1969). If electrocardiography shows the presence of two ventricular complexes on the standard limb leads in either twin this is diagnostic of ventricular independence. Cardiac catheterisation and angiography should be done if there is evidence of separate cardia and co-existing congenital heart disease. If there is a single ventricle, catheterisation is necessary to obtain anatomical and physiological data before separation can be contemplated (Nichols, Blattner and Rudolph, 1967).

Isotope-tagged albumin given into the scalp vein and detected over the posterior chest wall of each twin will show immediate exchange if there is common vasculature, and a delay of several minutes occurs if they are separate. Other techniques for studying cross-circulation include the injection of intravenous dyes such as indigo carmine (which is excreted in the urine), methylene blue and fluorescein, which, if injected into the common umbilical vein, colours the skin of one or both babies, depending on the degree of communication. Oral glucose tolerance tests and intravenous renographic dyes have also been used (Nichols, Blattner and Rudolph, 1967).

Straight x-rays of abdomen give limited information about gastrointestinal communications, and neither gallbladder may be outlined by an oral cholecystogram. Intravenous pyelography may demonstrate normality or otherwise of the urinary tracts (Simpson, 1969). Oral administration of dyes such as carmine red or brilliant cresyl blue to one infant results in the dye appearing in the stools of one or both twins. If the dye is excreted by both, radiological examination (using thin barium) is necessary to determine the site of conjunction, because of the possibility that the common bile duct may be involved, since all thoracopagus twins have a shared liver (Nichols, Blattner and Rudolph, 1967).

The timing of elective separation should take pulmonary maturity into account (Nichols, Blattner and Rudolph, 1967), and the optimum age is probably three months, when cardiopulmonary physiology is believed to be stabilised. On the other hand, emergency operation may be indicated soon after birth, either because of poor general condition, or because one twin is stillborn. Strict isolation from birth until the time of operation is advisable, to reduce the risks of infection. Preoperatively nasogastric suction helps to decompress the gastrointestinal tract (Simpson, 1969) and antibiotic cover, pre- and postoperatively, prevents intercurrent infection (Simpson, 1969; De Angelis, Dursi and Ibach, 1970). The physiological and biochemical functions which should be monitored before, during and after operation include body temperature, blood pressure, pulse rate, $P\text{CO}_2$, $P\text{O}_2$, urinary output, ECG and EEG. Femoral arterial and venous catheterisation permit arterial and central venous pressure measurements, which help in the maintenance of adequate ventilation and blood pressure during the operation. Because of difficulties in making an accurate swab and instrument count when two operations are being done simultaneously, postoperative x-ray ensures that none has been left in situ, and also may detect unsuspected pneumothorax (Simpson, 1969).

In true thoracopagus the sternum is always joined and this presents problems in skin closure. Undercutting the skin margins may increase intra-abdominal pressure to the point where respiratory embarrassment and impeded venous return to the heart occur (Nichols, Blattner and Rudolph, 1967; Simpson, 1969). This can be overcome by closing the abdominal defect temporarily with mesh and siliconised rubber, and skin grafting the defect at a later date (Simpson, 1969).

Postoperatively, continued monitoring and intensive care are necessary. Respiratory failure, apnoea and atelectasis may require endotracheal intubation and repeated suction to remove thick mucus secretions (De Angelis, Dursi and Ibach, 1970). Digitalisation may be needed if cardiac failure supervenes, especially if there is associated congenital heart disease (Simpson, 1969; De Angelis, Dursi and Ibach, 1970).

In cases of omphalopagus the timing of surgery is also elective, unless there was tissue damage at delivery and the omphalocoele ruptured, when emergency separation soon after birth should be considered. Repair of the umbilical defect only may be of value where further maturation may make surgery at a later date a more feasible proposition.

BIRTH TRAUMA

Birth trauma is only more common in multiple than singleton births because abnormal presentations are more common. Their symptomatology and treatment are no different, and probably the only ones of note are intracranial haemorrhage, because pre-term infants are particularly at risk, and fractures of the cervical spine due to hyperextension of the head in breech delivery.

Intracranial haemorrhage may be due to traumatic delivery or result from anoxia. Clinically there may be birth asphyxia, followed by episodes of apnoea, changes in muscle tone, a high pitched cry, increased fontanelle tension and convulsions. Lateralising signs are infrequent but may be found in some babies with subdural haematoma. Repeated subdural taps may prevent permanent brain damage in these cases, but subarachnoid, intraventricular and intracerebral haemorrhage can only be treated symptomatically. Whatever the site of the bleeding, the prognosis must be guarded for those who survive since only about 30 per cent of them will be normal and most of them will be severely handicapped (Natelson and Sayers, 1973).

Cervical fractures luckily are rare, since the prognosis is bad and the few who survive are left with paraplegia in extension. At birth the infant lies with arms abducted and with complete flaccid paralysis below the lesion. Permanent damage is not found in those born by Caesarean section, but is confined to those delivered vaginally (Abroms, Bresman and Zuckerman, 1973).

CONGENITAL MALFORMATIONS

Most mothers are worried that their children may be abnormal at birth and if one twin or triplet has some defect it is natural for the parents to think that the other(s) will be similarly affected, especially if they are identical. Although identical pairs are more likely to have some abnormality than fraternal pairs, each may be affected in a different way or to a different degree (Fogel, Nitowsky and Gruenwald, 1956; Francois, Van Leuvan and Vercanteren, 1972; Pembrey, 1972; Revesz, 1973). If an abnormality is present at birth the parents usually want to know if and when it can be corrected and if subsequent children will be born with the same defect.

Some of the more common defects, especially those needing attention in the neonatal period, will be discussed here, in relation to their inheritance and management.

CENTRAL NERVOUS SYSTEM

Some of these abnormalities are likely to be diagnosed antenatally in multiple pregnancy because these patients are often x-rayed before delivery, and the obstetrician is therefore more likely to become involved with the problem before the paediatrician.

Spina bifida cystica may have a racial basis but it is likely that social factors play a part in its aetiology (Lorber, 1972a). The risk of having a second affected baby is about one in 20 and this rises to one in eight if there are two affected children (*Human Genetics*, 1972). About ten per cent of cases are simple meningocoeles which are not associated with neurological involvement. There is no urgency to treat skin-covered lesions, but occipital meningocoeles and encephalocoeles should be referred for early surgery whatever the covering. In those with simple spinal defects the end result is good (Cook, 1971; Lorber, 1972a) but most children with meningomyelocoeles require repeated operations and highly skilled medical and para-medical care for the rest of their short lives. With no surgical intervention the mortality is 90 per cent in the first year. Early operation results in a survival rate of 49 per cent but two-thirds of these children will die by the time they are seven years old and the rest will not live beyond their early twenties (Mawdsley, Rickman and Roberts, 1967; Eckstein, 1968; Lorber, 1972a). If operation is contemplated it should be done as soon as possible, within 48 hours of birth if possible, to reduce the risk of meningitis, but the decision to close the defect should depend not only on the extent of the abnormality but also on the home conditions, the parents' attitude to the situation, and their ability to cope with a potentially severely handicapped child (Lorber, 1972b).

Hydrocephalus. Apart from the rare sex-linked type, found only in males, there is no known genetic basis for uncomplicated hydrocephalus. Isolated hydrocephalus requires early investigation to differentiate it from hydrancephaly, which is inoperable, but treatment is not urgent unless the head is enlarging rapidly. The majority of cases will arrest spontaneously, but treatment by head wrapping (Epstein, Hochwald and Ransohoff, 1973) or oral isosorbide (Lorber, 1972c) may have a temporary but favourable effect, and postpone or prevent operation. Spitz–Holter and Pudenz–Heyer shunts give good results if there is no spina bifida (Van der Veen, 1972), but uncomplicated hydrocephalus is uncommon, 80 per cent of those with hydrocephalus also having meningomyelocoele and 80 per cent of those with meningomyelocoele also having hydrocephalus. Even though 50 per cent of treated hydrocephalics have a normal I.Q., many are severely retarded or spastic (Cook, 1971).

GASTROINTESTINAL SYSTEM

Cleft lip and palate may occur separately or together and they have a partial and complex inheritance (Hanart and Kalin, 1972). The risk of being born with this deformity is about one in 30 for the children and siblings of affected persons, but if a parent with a cleft lip already has one affected child, the risk to further children rises to about one in ten (*Human Genetics*, 1972). Surgical treatment is not usually undertaken in the neonatal period, but pre-operative splinting leads to more satisfactory cosmetic results. Surprisingly few infants have feeding problems, but those who do need specialised nursing care. Cleft lip is repaired when the baby is three months old and the palate closed at about nine months, before the baby starts to babble.

Oesophageal atresia. Multiple pregnancy is often associated with polyhydramnios and polyhydramnios is also significant in relation to high intestinal obstruction in the fetus, in particular oesophageal atresia. This is not a true familial defect, but genetic factors may play a part in its pathogenesis (Schinke, Leape and Holder, 1972). It can occur in more than one child in a family, in mother and child as well as in both twins (Young and Drainer, 1972). The diagnosis should always be considered in a twin pregnancy where there is hydramnios and one baby is much smaller than the other. Immediate treatment is necessary, and pre-operatively these babies need intravenous fluids, repeated pharyngeal suction and perhaps endotracheal intubation and artificial ventilation. In ten per cent of cases there is no tracheo-oesophageal fistula, but if the gap between the proximal and distal ends is wide, preliminary oesophagostomy and gastrostomy is preferable to immediate end-to-end anastomosis. Postoperatively their progress depends on the type of abnormality, birthweight and the presence of other abnormalities. About 25 per cent of them have cardiac defects and other gastrointestinal or respiratory anomalies may also be present (Young and Drainer, 1972).

Other anatomical (as opposed to functional) obstructions are uncommon and they too require treatment as soon as they are diagnosed. Most neonates withstand operative procedures remarkably well in the first few days of life, if their general condition is good and there are no added complications.

Diaphragmatic hernia may present the obstetrician with resuscitation problems, the baby remaining cyanosed and dyspnoeic despite endotracheal oxygen. Operative treatment is urgent in severe cases, and many of these babies die because they also have hypoplastic lungs and other abnormalities. The outlook is good if the symptoms are mild, or only become apparent after 24 hours of age.

CARDIOVASCULAR SYSTEM

The most common cardiac malformations are septal defects and patent ductus arteriosus. About one per cent are due to a single mutant gene, four per cent to chromosomal defects and the rest to multifactorial inheritance (Nora and Spangler, 1972). In general, there is a one in 30 recurrence risk when one child is already known to have a defect, but the recurrence rates for each particular type of defect are not known (*Human Genetics*, 1972). Advanced techniques have made it possible to diagnose congenital heart disease in the first few days of life, but many of them do not need treatment or detailed investigation until they are older. Surgical treatment may be corrective or palliative, depending on the type of malformation, and the most common postoperative complications are heart failure and acid–base disturbances (Stark, 1972). The neonatal mortality varies from 50 to 90 per cent, depending on the type of abnormality (Campbell, 1973).

OTHER MALFORMATIONS

Club foot is said to be more common in multiple pregnancies (see Chapter 12) and talipes equinovarus is more common than talipes calcaneo valgus. Most cases of true deformity are corrected by manipulation and strapping. Relapses or failures of conservative management may need surgical soft tissue release at about 12 weeks old, and any residual deformity when the child is three years old requires further operative repair. There is an increased risk (about one in fifty) that subsequent children may also have talipes equinovarus (*Human Genetics*, 1972).

Congenital dislocation of the hip occurs in utero, probably in the last few weeks before term, and is more common in breech deliveries. Although babies of less than 1700 g often have unstable hips, true dislocation is uncommon (Barlow, 1968). Because of their immaturity and malpresentation multiple births are likely to have 'clicking hips' on abduction, but most of them will recover spontaneously. Those who still have joint laxity when they are a week old must be treated by keeping the hips in full abduction with a simple plastic splint, which fits over the nappy. If treatment is started early enough recovery is complete and more prolonged and painful treatment can be avoided. Both genetic and environmental factors play a part in its aetiology and the recurrence risk is one in 40 for brothers and sons and one in 10 for sisters and daughters (*Human Genetics*, 1972).

Genetic counselling is essential whenever an inherited defect has occurred and the parents often worry less if the chances of another child being affected are explained to them. If a twin (or higher multiple) is found to have an abnormality, it is essential that his sibling(s) are examined thoroughly not only for the defect in question, but also for any other abnormality.

PROBLEMS OF THE LOW BIRTHWEIGHT BABY

The problems of the low birthweight baby vary according to his gestational age, and they have been outlined by Davies and his colleagues (1972) as follows:

Pre-term	Term
Respiratory problems:	Respiratory problems:
Hyaline membrane disease	Severe birth asphyxia
Apnoeic attacks	Pulmonary haemorrhage
	'Pneumonia'
Inability to suck or swallow	Symptomatic hypoglycaemia
Hypothermia	Hypothermia
Jaundice	Polycythaemia
Infection	Intrauterine viral infection:
	Rubella
	Cytomegalovirus
Functional intestinal obstruction	Congenital abnormalities
Necrotising enterocolitis	

Babies who are both pre-term and small-for-dates may have a combination of any of these problems.

Respiratory problems may vary from being so slight and transient that they require little or no treatment, to being so severe that they need the full neo-natal armamentarium of radiological, physiological and biochemical moni-toring, intravenous therapy and mechanical ventilation, not to mention experienced nursing and observation. This intensive care may have to be continued for several days, and the end result depends on the cause of the respiratory difficulty and the occurrence of complications such as apnoeic attacks and cerebral or pulmonary haemorrhage.

Hypoglycaemia is common in those who are small-for-dates and the smaller twin (especially if his weight is much below that of his sibling) is particularly vulnerable. All babies at risk should be screened daily by pre-feed Dextrostix for the first three days and levels of less than 25 mg per cent need to be checked by a blood glucose estimation. Early feeding reduces the risk of hypoglycaemia and prevention is better than cure, especially as those who develop symptoms may suffer permanent brain damage (Koivisto, Sequerios and Kranse, 1972).

Neonatal jaundice. Because of less efficient glucuronidation, the pre-term infant is liable to develop severe and prolonged hyperbilirubinaemia, even in the absence of blood group incompatibilities, and phototherapy is indicated once the indirect bilirubin level has reached 15 mg per cent or more. Since these infants need their eyes covered as long as treatment lasts, it is important that they are examined before, during and after treatment, otherwise it can be difficult to determine the aetiology of any eye defects detected later. Exchange transfusion may be needed if the bilirubin rises to 20 mg per cent, or even at lower levels if the baby is very immature or has suffered from hypoxia, either of which might predispose to kernicterus. In a six-year follow-up, Culley, Powell and Waterhouse (1970) found that neurological handicap was limited to those of low birthweight, and not directly related to the depth of jaundice. There was no lowering of intelligence in those with non-haemolytic disease if their bilirubin had not exceeded 20 mg per cent.

FEEDING

Full-term twins and triplets, who weigh more than 2500 g can be fed the same as any other normal baby. Four-hourly feeds of breast milk or full-strength half-cream dried milk can be started as soon as possible, the baby being allowed to take as much (or as little) as he wants at each feed. Obviously with more than one baby, especially if they are born early, breast feeding has its problems but it is worth remembering that some of the qualities of breast milk enable the newborn to withstand infection (Hanson and Winberg, 1972) and in underdeveloped countries it is also a defence against iatrogenic malnutrition. Very small or ill infants need smaller, more frequent concentrated feeds and if they are unable to suck or swallow may have to be tube fed. Low birthweight babies need iron and vitamin supplements such as 5 ml half-strength Sytron (sodium ironedetate) daily, starting at four weeks old and continuing until they are weaned. Vitamin drops, such as Abidec, 0.3 ml daily, can be started at ten days old, and given by spoon or dropper before a feed.

CONTINUING CARE

Small babies may spend several weeks in the special nursery, but if there are no additional complications they can usually go home when their weight reaches 2250 to 2500 g depending on the home circumstances and the prevailing weather. Small babies often come from poor homes and (particularly in the case of multiple births) it is important to make sure that the mother can cope with the extra babies. If not, the appropriate welfare services should be informed before the babies go home. In any case the mother should be told about the need for warmth, the dangers of infection and the importance of iron and vitamin supplements.

Not all babies who have had special neonatal care need to be seen again by the hospital staff, and the timing of any return visits will depend largely on local practice and the reason for the follow-up. If the mother is told the reason why the baby must be seen again, she is more likely to keep the appointment.

SUMMARY

Practically all the problems encountered by multiple births in the neonatal period are the same as those for singletons of the same weight and gestation. Their survival depends on the supervision, experience and close liaison of a well-trained, well-equipped nursing, medical and para-medical team, with the backing of the social services once the babies go home. For many of them their problems will have been solved by the time they go home, but for others they might only be beginning. The care they receive in the first few weeks of life should be such that their handicaps are lessened, not aggravated, and their parents helped and not burdened with unnecessary difficulties.

CHAPTER 14

Prognosis for the Babies, Early and Late

V. FARR

People have always been fascinated by multiple births and primitive societies have differed in their attitudes towards them, in many cases believing that they were the result of evil spirits or (more mundanely) of infidelity. In either case the outlook for the babies was poor, since more often than not they were killed or left to die. Even in these days of more enlightened aetiological views the babies of multiple pregnancies have a poorer than average chance of survival since their intrauterine existence is hazardous and they are more vulnerable to the difficulties of birth and more likely to be handicapped when they get older. Unfortunately the interest that their lifespan engenders in the English-speaking medical literature is much more in favour of twins rather than higher multiples. Although the first specific reference to quadruplets was made by Hagedorn in 1685 (quoted by Hamilton, Brown and Spiers, 1959) very little, apart from individual case reports, has been written about the prognosis for triplets and quadruplets, especially in the last 20 years. Since most of these reports are concerned with those pregnancies where the babies survived, they are of no value in assessing overall prognosis. This chapter is therefore mainly concerned with twin pregnancy but it is reasonable to suppose that much of the information is equally relevant to other multiple pregnancies, since triplets, quadruplets and quintuplets are only variations and combinations of one- and two-egg twins (Miettinen, 1954; Miettinen and Grönroos, 1956). Where data are available on triplets and higher multiples they have, of course, been included.

MORTALITY RATES

In 1962 MacDonald reported a series of 500 consecutive twin deliveries in Glasgow. The gross perinatal mortality, including infants born alive before

188

28 weeks gestation, was 12.5 per cent, but widely different rates have been quoted, e.g. 28.1 per cent (Munnell and Taylor, 1946), 14 per cent (Potter and Fuller, 1949), 11 per cent (Bender, 1952), 9.2 per cent (Little and Friedman, 1958), and 12.3 per cent (Tow, 1959). A more recent report (Patten, 1970) of 1001 multiple births gave a perinatal mortality rate of 12.5 per cent in twins and 18.8 per cent in higher multiples, compared with 4.8 per cent for all births.

Unfortunately it is difficult to compare the results of different series as many factors, apart from selection criteria, influence the outcome of pregnancy, such as differences in socioeconomic conditions, facilities for antenatal care, obstetric training and expertise, and the incidence of complications. Even so, it is clear that these infants have a much poorer chance of survival than singletons, not only in the perinatal period but also in the first year of life (Barr and Stevenson, 1961) and the greater the number of fetuses the greater the hazards (Leading Article, *British Medical Journal*, 1968). It is worth remembering that mortality rates do not convey that more than one baby is at risk since the proportion of twin pregnancies which ends in disaster for one or both babies may be as high as one in six (Dunn, 1965) and the outlook is even worse for triplet and quadruplet pregnancies (Miettinen, 1954).

Twin perinatal loss is at least three times that of singletons (Anderson, 1956; Potter, 1963; Butler and Alberman, 1969) and is even greater for triplets and quads (Beacham and Beacham, 1950; Miettinen, 1954; Kurtz, Davies and Loftus, 1958), and is due mainly to neonatal rather than prenatal deaths. The stillbirth rate is about twice as high in twins as in single births, about three times as high in triplets and four times as high in quads (Bulmer, 1970). In the first month of life differences in mortality are even greater, being about five times higher in twins and almost twenty times higher in triplets when compared to singletons. These differences become less marked with increasing age, until by the second year mortality rates are the same (Bulmer, 1970). Anderson (1956) showed that the prognosis for liveborn twins improved considerably in the years 1938 to 1952, largely because of improved paediatric care, but the stillbirth rate showed no consistent improvement over the same period. The same trend is found in the literature covering the past 25 to 30 years. Neonatal mortality amongst twins has fallen from around 20 per cent to less than 10 per cent, a difference of tenfold to twofold when compared to singletons, whereas the stillbirth rate has only varied from about 3.5 to 5.5 per cent, which is two to three times that for singletons (Anderson, 1957; Little and Friedman, 1958; Potter, 1963; Dunn, 1965). The perinatal death rate for triplets has also fallen considerably since the beginning of this century (Beacham and Beacham, 1950) and the prognosis for triplets and quadruplets in Finland showed a gradual improvement over the years 1905 to 1952 (Miettinen, 1954). Although only 14 of the 72 quadruplets in this series survived, in the previous century all four babies rarely if ever survived, and the earliest recorded success in this respect was quadruplets born in 1915 (Hamilton, Brown and Spiers, 1959). Needless to say, quintuplet survival is even rarer, and by 1968 only four sets were known to have survived (Leading Article, *British Medical Journal*, 1968).

Many factors affect the prognosis for these babies, and they will now be considered in more detail.

MATERNAL FACTORS

AGE

There are contradictory views on how much maternal age affects twin mortality. Karn (1953) found that the mothers of non-survivors, especially when both babies died, were much younger than the mothers of twins who survived. In her series the mean age of mothers with two live infants was 31.8 years, compared to 26.5 years for mothers who lost both babies. In the 1958 British Perinatal Mortality Survey (Butler and Alberman, 1969) the babies at greatest risk were those whose mothers were under 20 years old. These mothers have an almost one in five chance of losing both infants. On the other hand, this survey showed that increasing age does not have the adverse effect on perinatal mortality that it has in singleton pregnancies. In contradiction, Barr and Stevenson (1961) found that there was no relationship between maternal age and fetal death and Parsons (1964), in a study of unlike-sex pairs, came to the same conclusion.

It is possible that selection factors account for these differences. Karn's figures are based on hospital data and the Perinatal Survey included all deaths in the United Kingdom over a three-month period. Both these studies based their results on deaths from 28 weeks' gestation to the first month after birth. Barr and Stevenson analysed stillbirths and first year deaths occurring in all legitimate births in England and Wales and these mothers were on average a year older than the mothers of singletons born in the same year, but about two years younger than the mothers in Karn's study. Parson's series consisted of dizygotic (DZ) twins who were either stillborn or died before going home from hospital. Of the 265 mothers only 15 were under 21.

In a review of locked twins six of the 37 mothers were over 30 years old, and the perinatal mortality in this group was 20 per cent compared to 40.9 per cent for those born to mothers younger than this (Khunda, 1972).

PARITY

There is no doubt that twins born to primigravidae have a poorer chance of survival than those born subsequently, the overall mortality in first pregnancies being between 16 and 18 per cent (Farrell, 1964; Klein, 1964; Parsons, 1964). This represents a loss two or three times greater than that for subsequent pregnancies, despite the fact that about four times as many babies are born to multigravidae. This increased risk holds true even when taking into account fetal malformation and babies weighing less than 1 kg (Klein, 1964). Law (1967) analysed 1567 twin and nine triplet pregnancies born between 1962 and 1964. Although the overall mortality was low (8.1 per cent) it was higher in primiparae (10 per cent) than multiparae (7.3 per cent). When macerated stillbirths, and those with malformations incompatible with life were excluded the corrected rates were 6.6, 8.5 and 5.7 per cent respectively. In locked twins, perinatal mortality falls from 27.5 per cent in first pregnancies to 10 per cent in higher parities (Khunda, 1972).

Although there is no significant difference in mean parity for survivors and non-survivors in general, both twins are more likely to die if they come at the beginning of the family (Karn, 1953). After the first pregnancy there is no consistent correlation between individual parities and mortality (Farrell, 1964) but there is a slight increase in perinatal loss in higher parities, but this does not reach the levels found in primigravidae (Parsons, 1964; Butler and Alberman, 1969).

MATERNAL HEIGHT

Anderson (1956) found that the perinatal mortality for babies weighing between three and five pounds (1.4 to 2.3 kg) was three times greater for short women than for tall. This difference was not found for babies of less than three pounds, and so few of the bigger babies died that the numbers were insufficient to make valid comparison. As a group, tall women produce large babies and their ability to cope with the demands of carrying more than one baby may be the result of better health, nutrition and physique.

SOCIAL CLASS

As with maternal height, little has been written on the effect of social class on the outcome of multiple pregnancy. In a study of prematurely born children, Alm (1953) found that lower social class had a more deleterious effect on low birthweight twins than on singletons of the same weight or on heavier controls. This study was restricted to legitimate male infants, born in hospital, so the conclusions drawn from it may not be applicable to the general population.

PREGNANCY COMPLICATIONS

PRE-ECLAMPTIC TOXAEMIA

Multiple pregnancy carries an increased risk of pregnancy complications, especially pre-eclampsia which occurs in about 20 to 30 per cent of cases (Anderson, 1956; Farrell, 1964). However, perinatal mortality may be as high, or even higher, in those patients with no complications at all (Anderson, 1956) and toxaemia is not the major contributor to fetal mortality that it is in singletons (Spurway, 1962). Anderson (1956) found that although mortality increased with the severity of the disease, severe pre-eclampsia and eclampsia accounted for less than ten per cent of all deaths, and the overall mortality in those with toxaemia was half that found in those with no pregnancy complications. Although one-third of mothers with twins had some degree of toxaemia only one-fifth of the baby deaths occurred in this group. Farrell (1964) came to the same conclusion and he thought that the reduced mortality was due to the mothers in his study receiving hospital care and bed rest before delivery. Another explanation may be that many pregnancies terminate early, before symptoms of toxaemia become evident.

PREMATURE ONSET OF LABOUR

Although most women who are having twins have no antenatal complications whatsoever, most authors agree that prematurity, whether based on weight or gestation, is one of the most important factors contributing to the high perinatal mortality in multiple pregnancy. Fetal loss increases with decreasing gestation and over 50 per cent of twins born five weeks or more before term do not survive (Robertson, 1964; Dunn, 1965). The majority of neonatal deaths are in this group (Sherman and Lowe, 1970) and although they are often of average weight-for-dates, it is usual for both babies to die. On the other hand most stillbirths are delivered after the 35th week and rarely do both babies die in utero. These infants are generally small-for-dates, and even the surviving baby is smaller than expected (Dunn, 1965). Twins born long before term have a better chance of survival than singletons of the same gestation, but after 37 weeks the converse is true. This is particularly so for second twins whose death rates, compared to singletons, rise steeply in late pregnancy. As far as survival is concerned, the best time for first twins to be born is 39 weeks gestation, and for second twins 37 to 38 weeks, which suggests that multiple pregnancies of 40 weeks and more should be considered to be postmature (Dunn, 1965; Butler and Alberman, 1969).

ABORTION

Information about multiple pregnancies which terminate before 20 weeks' gestation is inevitably incomplete and therefore data which are available are not absolutely reliable, but it does seem that they are no more liable to abort at this time than singletons (Benirschke and Driscoll, 1967). There is, however, an increased risk of abortion between 24 and 28 weeks, which may be due to differences in zygosity (since more monozygotic than dizygotic pairs are born at this time) but may also be due to placentation, since Naeye and his colleagues (1966) have shown that more than twice as many monochorial as dichorial twin pregnancies end in late abortion.

HYDRAMNIOS

Hydramnios in multiple pregnancy is a poor prognostic sign since it is often associated with premature delivery or gross fetal malformation. Mortality may be as high as 41 per cent, but varies with the degree of excess liquor, the more severe forms being associated with death from prematurity (Anderson, 1956).

OTHER ANTENATAL COMPLICATIONS

Other complications of multiple pregnancy in relation to their effect on perinatal mortality are reported so infrequently that their significance cannot be assessed.

HOSPITALISATION

The effect of hospitalisation on perinatal mortality has not yet been satisfactorily evaluated, and the pros and cons of antenatal admission have been discussed fully in Chapter 9.

LABOUR AND DELIVERY

PRESENTATION AND MODE OF DELIVERY

There is an increased incidence of malpresentation in multiple pregnancy and about two-thirds of deliveries need operative assistance (Tow, 1959). Fetal mortality increases rapidly when presentation is other than vertex (Aaron, Silverman and Halperin, 1961) though in babies weighing less than 4 lb (1.8 kg) the mortality is high even after spontaneous vertex delivery. In the very immature baby, size is of far greater importance than the method of delivery in determining his chance of survival (Anderson, 1956). Malpresentation is much more common in second-born twins and plays a considerable part in the increased risk for this twin (Farrell, 1964). It seems likely that malpresentation is an even greater problem for triplets and higher multiples but no information is available on how much this contributes to their high death rates.

Just how much risk is involved with the different types of delivery is debatable and to some extent must depend on the skill and experience of the operator, but it is reckoned that about a quarter of multiple births are liable to birth trauma as a result of breech extraction or forceps delivery through an inadequately dilated cervix (Dunn, 1965). The highest mortality is found in spontaneous unattended breech delivery (Aaron, Silverman and Halperin, 1961; Farrell, 1964), the risks being greater for the first than for the second twin (Aaron, Silverman and Halperin, 1961; Butler and Alberman, 1969). On the other hand Anderson (1956) considered that the method of delivery had little or no effect on perinatal mortality except for babies of between 4 and 5.5 lb (1.8 to 2.5 kg) who, after internal version, were delivered by breech extraction; and even in these cases other factors such as fetal distress and prolapsed cord may have contributed to the high stillbirth rate. Klein

(1964) found virtually no difference in mortality between vertex and breech presentations, and in fact, if antepartum deaths and babies of less than 1.0 kg were excluded, fetal loss was higher in those presenting by the vertex. These results, however, are unusual and any form of operative delivery, especially when associated with manipulative procedures, is usually detrimental to the baby's welfare.

The most lethal forms of delivery are spontaneous breech delivery and breech extraction (with or without preceding podalic version) (Kurtz, Davis and Loftus, 1958; Aaron, Silverman and Halperin, 1961; Farrell, 1964; Leading Article, *British Medical Journal*, 1968) and the prognosis is even worse for small babies, the hazards of breech delivery increasing rapidly with decreasing birthweight. The excessive loss found in all types of breech delivery can be explained by the large number of very small babies who present by the breech (Little and Friedman, 1958). The safest forms of delivery are spontaneous vertex (whether or not preceded by cephalic version), low forceps delivery and Caesarean section (Aaron, Silverman and Halperin, 1961; Farrell, 1964; Dunn, 1965).

DELIVERY INTERVAL

Undue haste in delivering the babies carries a poorer prognosis than prolonged delays. Excluding those cases where a rapid delivery is unavoidable, e.g. prolapsed cord, the mortality is higher (16.3 per cent) when the delivery interval is less than ten minutes compared to delays of more than 20 minutes, when mortality is 13.5 per cent (Farrell, 1964). However, this does not mean that the second baby should wait too long, even though a case is recorded of a delay of 35 days, and the twin survived (Abrams, 1957). The optimum time between deliveries is between ten and twenty minutes, the fetal loss being about half that found when delivery occurs outwith these limits (Farrell, 1964). Over 95 per cent of deaths following vaginal delivery occur when the interval is less than 10 minutes (Klein, 1964) but in cases where only the second twin dies, 61 per cent are born more than thirty minutes after the surviving twin, compared to 21 per cent where the second baby is the only survivor (Butler and Alberman, 1969). Second twins born between 2.5 and 15 minutes after the first have the same uncorrected mortality as their co-twins. This is the result of management of labour which involves neither excessive speed nor undue delay in completing the delivery, and applies equally to triplet delivery (Kurtz, Davis and Loftus, 1958). In this group increased survival is found in all types of delivery, but the safest way out for the second twin is spontaneous vertex delivery 10 to 15 minutes after his sibling (Tow, 1959; Spurway, 1962). The poorest outlook is for those delivered by breech extraction after a delay of less than 5 or more than 25 minutes. The type of delivery makes little difference to fetal wastage when the delay between births is prolonged (Little and Friedman, 1958).

OTHER COMPLICATIONS OF LABOUR

Anaesthesia

A large number of multiple births will need some form of anaesthesia during labour or at the time of delivery. Saddle block and spinal anaesthesia do not affect mortality rates and nitrous oxide also appears to be safe in most cases, but the second twin (for no obvious reason) often fares badly with caudal or epidural anaesthesia as well as with prolonged inhalation anaesthesia (Little and Friedman, 1958). The injudicious use of anaesthesia is also just as detrimental to triplets (Kurtz, Davis and Loftus, 1958). However, in a later series the second twin fared better than the first, despite an operative rate of 80 per cent. This was attributed to the use of conduction anaesthesia which did not have the depressant effect of inhalation agents, and also seemed to be superior not only to local anaesthesia but also to no anaesthesia at all (Aaron, Silverman and Halperin, 1961). Presumably this was due to improved maternal relaxation with a subsequently less traumatic delivery.

Locked twins

This rare condition has been discussed earlier (page 160). The most common form of presentation is first twin breech and second twin vertex. Mortality is high, especially for the first twin (about 65 per cent) and nearly a third of all locked twins do not survive the delivery (Khunda, 1972).

Conjoined twins

Luckily this is an even rarer event than locked twins, for the survival rate is extremely low. More often than not the diagnosis is made at the time of delivery, when there is probably no alternative to destructive operation. If the condition is discovered earlier, Caesarean section gives the babies a better chance of survival (also see page 172). Under ideal conditions the commonest form (thoracopagus) has a good chance of successful operative separation and the babies can develop normally, but in general their prognosis is poor (Tan et al, 1971a).

FETAL FACTORS

FETAL SEX

Perinatal mortality is affected not only by the sex of the individual baby but also by the sex of the twin pairs. Unlike-sex pairs have a better chance of survival than like-sex pairs (Potter, 1963; Klein, 1964; Dunn, 1965) and girls do better than boys (Barr and Stevenson, 1961; Spurway, 1962; Potter,

1963). Boys are responsible for the higher mortality in like-sex pairs (Myrianthopoulos, 1970); more male pairs die before 28 weeks than like-sex female pairs (Barr and Stevenson, 1961), and almost twice as many boys die in the neonatal period compared to the number who are stillborn. On the other hand, twin girls are more likely to be born dead than to die in the first week (Klein, 1964). The highest mortality is found in like-sex twin boys where almost one in ten pregnancies ends in the death of both babies, whereas in like-sex female pairs the death of both babies is less common than in any other group (Butler and Alberman, 1969) and the lowest death rates are found in the girls of unlike-sex pairs (Barr and Stevenson, 1961). Boys have a better chance of survival if the co-twin is a girl rather than another boy (Potter, 1963). The perinatal loss for male–male pairs is 15.9 per cent, for male–female pairs 14.4 per cent and for female–female pairs 11.4 per cent. Twins of the same sex and blood group have the poorest chance of survival and those of different sex and different blood groups the best prognosis (Potter, 1963).

Mortality rates in the first year of life follow much the same pattern as perinatal deaths, boys being at greater risk than girls. An analysis of perinatal mortality for male twins and female twins in the same pregnancies by Donaldson and Kohl (1965) showed that although the fetal death rates were the same, the neonatal loss was significantly higher for the males. Both like- and opposite-sex twins have similar chances that one of them will die in the first year, but once one has died there is a greater chance that the other will die too if they are of the same sex, especially if they are also monozygotic (MZ). When both babies die before their first birthday, like-sex pairs are more likely to die at about the same age than those of unlike-sex (Barr and Stevenson, 1961).

ZYGOSITY

The difference in mortality between like- and unlike-sex pairs is probably due to the number of MZ twins among those of like sex, since the loss of MZ pairs is two to three times that of DZ pairs (Potter, 1963; Myriantho-poulos, 1970). Assuming that the survival of the individuals of DZ pairs is not influenced in utero by the sex of the co-twin, estimations of fetal loss and deaths within the first year show that the rates are higher for MZ than DZ pairs, regardless of sex, even though the risks are higher for boys than girls (Barr and Stevenson, 1961). On this basis zygosity may also play a part in the high fetal loss in triplets and quadruplets, although on the small amount of information available it has been estimated that very few of them are monozygotic (MZ). Miettinen (1954), in a review of the literature, came to the conclusion that MZ triplets are the rarest of the possible combinations, but MZ quintuplets may be more frequent than is generally believed (Newman, 1942).

One or both twins die in 16.4 per cent of MZ pregnancies, whereas an unfavourable outcome is found in only 5.3 per cent of cases where the babies are dizygotic (DZ) (Potter, 1963). Twins that share the same fate, i.e.

both die or both survive, are usually monozygotic (MZ) (Karn, 1953) although with the exception of prematurity, which is more common in MZ twins, the cause of death may not be related to zygosity.

PLACENTATION

MZ pairs with monochorionic placentas have the highest death rates and unlike-sex DZ pairs with separate placentas have the lowest. The perinatal death rate in Gruenwald's (1970) series was 7.1 per cent in monochorionic pairs, 4.6 per cent in dichorionic pairs of the same sex and 3.6 per cent in dichorionic pairs of the opposite sex. In another study, Myrianthopoulos (1970) showed that fetal loss was highest amongst monoamniotic mono-chorionic twins (22.2 per cent) and lowest in those who were diamniotic and dichorionic (3.9 per cent) whereas neonatal deaths were highest in the diamniotic monochorionic pairs (13.7 per cent) and lowest in the mono-amniotic monochorionic pairs (5.6 per cent). The overall perinatal death rate was 27.8 per cent for those who were monoamniotic monochorionic, 22.5 per cent for twins who were diamniotic monochorionic and 10.9 per cent for the diamniotic dichorionic pairs.

Vascular transplacental anastomoses and inequality in the size of the placentas play an important part in this high fetal wastage, together with other factors such as cord entanglement and placental insufficiency (Wharton, Edwards and Cameron, 1968). Monoamniotic, monochorionic twins are born earlier and weigh less than others and also show a higher incidence of birthweight disparity. Their stillbirth rate is almost twice that for diamniotic monochorionic twins and a third of them die in the perinatal period. Only about half these pregnancies result in two live babies (Wharton, Edwards and Cameron, 1968).

BIRTH ORDER

Although first-born twins fare much the same as singletons of the same weight, their co-twins do not, and most authors agree that the second twin (and the second and third triplet) has the poorer prognosis (Beacham and Beacham, 1950; Kurtz, Davis and Loftus, 1958; Little and Friedman, 1958; Klein, 1964; Butler and Alberman, 1969). Even excluding those of less than 1.0 kg, macerated stillbirths and those with malformations, the perinatal loss is at least one and one-half times that of first-borns (Guttmacher and Kohl, 1958; Spurway, 1962; Potter, 1963; Law, 1967).

In Ferguson's (1964) series there were 69.6 perinatal deaths per 1000 first babies and 115.5 for second babies, compared to a perinatal loss of 21.9 for singleton births. The most recently reported series (Patten, 1970) also confirmed that the perinatal mortality for later born infants was fifty per cent higher than for first-borns. On the other hand, Aaron and his colleagues (1961) did not find that this was so, and they thought that the second twin did better because of conduction anaesthesia and prompt delivery of the second baby. Bender (1952) and Potter and Fuller (1949) also considered that there was no increased risk to the second twin, and Chassar Moir (1964) said there was no increased stillbirth rate among second twins in Oxford. Graves and co-workers (Graves, Adams and Schreier, 1962) reported that the perinatal loss in second twins was less than in first, but their series was limited to primigravidae.

Most authors before 1960 agreed that the perinatal mortality was fifty per cent higher in second- compared to first-twin deliveries. In 1963 Wyshak and White reviewed the literature on the survival of twins and they found that in 23 594 infants the perinatal mortality was 57.1 per thousand for first-born and 74.6 per thousand for second-born twins. In only two of the series in this review (those of Aaron, Silverman and Halperin, 1961 and Romanowsky, 1962) were first twin deaths greater than those of the second twin.

It cannot be doubted that the risk to the second baby is much greater and suggestions that the birth hazard was non-existent, or only slightly increased, have come from workers reporting small series. Antepartum deaths are five times as common as in singletons (in first twins, twice as common). Second twins dying before the onset of labour do so about two weeks later than firstborn, suggesting that either they are at greater risk as pregnancy continues or that the death of the first twin is more likely to precipitate the onset of labour (Butler and Alberman, 1969). Another possible explanation is that when only one baby survives the dead twin takes second place at the time of delivery.

Intrapartum death and death due to trauma and anoxia during labour are more than twice as likely in first twins and four times as common in second twins compared to singletons, though it is unusual for both babies to die as a result of labour, except in pregnancies of very short duration (Butler and Alberman, 1969). Although second twins are more likely to die before delivery than in the neonatal period (Butler and Alberman, 1969; Myrianthopoulos, 1970) their stillbirth rate is much the same as that of first-born twins, but their neonatal death rate is twice as high (Little and Friedman, 1958; Sherman and Lowe, 1970). Many intrapartum and early postpartum deaths occur in cases where the delivery interval has been either too long or too short, or where there has been prolapse of the cord or early separation of the placenta (Anderson, 1956). It has been suggested that these complications put the second baby at risk of cerebral anoxia, whereas the first baby runs more danger of birth injury because he has to dilate the cervix (Potter, 1963). Apart from the possible reduction in uterine volume after delivery of the first baby, with consequent reduction in placental blood flow, other factors affecting mortality are malpresentation, operative delivery and prolapsed cord (Spurway, 1962; Farrell, 1964).

Over 200 years ago William Smellie (1752) noted that "The child that lies next to the fundus is the smallest and follows after the birth of the other, sometimes dead and putrified and sometimes in an emaciated condition" and the majority of third-born triplets are also the smallest of the litter (Miettinen and Grönroos, 1965). Because these babies are often smaller than their siblings one might expect them to have a higher death rate for this reason alone, but birthweight is not of such fundamental importance in determining their prognosis as it is for overall twin mortality, and the method of delivery of the second twin is more often than not the determining factor (Little and Friedman, 1958).

The second baby is at even greater risk when multiple pregnancy is undiagnosed at the time of delivery, since he may be trapped in utero or expelled too rapidly after the mother has been given oxytocin following the first infant's birth. Marked discrepancy in birthweight aggravates this situation, for if the first twin is large the fact that there is another baby to come is more likely to be missed. If the second twin is large, then there is the increased risk of birth trauma or asphyxia particularly if there is also malpresentation and the cervix is no longer dilated.

In opposite-sex pairs, where the second twin is a boy, the overall risk of his death is twice that of his sister's, but when the girl is second-born, her chances are the same as her brother's (Butler and Alberman, 1969). In monoamniotic pairs the number of survivors is small, but there is no obvious relationship between birth order and prognosis (Wharton, Edwards and Cameron, 1968).

Cerebral haemorrhage and birth asphyxia seem to occur with almost equal frequency in both first and second twins and the only conditions found more often in second-born babies are hyaline membrane disease and pneumonia. These are responsible for six times as many deaths in second as in first twins (Potter, 1963), and they seem to account for many of the differences in mortality associated with birth order.

BIRTHWEIGHT

It is to be expected that multiple pregnancy creates extra demands on the maternal supply system with consequent growth retardation of one or more babies. Although infants of short gestation are usually of average size for dates, those born later are often small (Dunn, 1965), reflecting the inadequacy of the placenta to maintain optimum nutritional supplies.

Low birthweight infants account for over 50 per cent of multiple births, compared to less than 10 per cent for singleton pregnancies (Potter, 1963) and birthweight is the most important single factor affecting the survival of multiple births (Karn, 1953; Miettinen, 1954; Klein, 1964). Mortality increases with decreasing birthweight and the excess mortality in multiple births is due mainly to the high incidence of very small babies of 1.0 kg or less, most of whom are so immature that they are incapable of independent existence (Aaron, Silverman and Halperin, 1961; Klein, 1964). None of the quadruplets in Miettinen's series (1954) weighed more than 2.5 kg and all those of less than 1.0 kg died within the first year.

With birthweights of over 2.5 kg, twin mortality is similar to that of singletons, and between 1.0 kg and 2.5 kg mortality is twice that of singletons (Potter, 1963). Twins weighing less than 2.5 kg have a fourfold chance of dying compared to twins who weigh more than this (Farrell, 1964; Robertson, 1964). There is a dramatic threefold improvement in survival once the 1.5 kg level is reached and a further significant change at 2.5 kg, with an overall critical level for survival around 2.0 kg (Guttmacher and Kohl, 1958; Farrell, 1964). Compared to singletons, whose optimum weight is between 3.5 and 4.0 kg, that for twins is between 2.5 and 3.5 kg (Butler and Alberman, 1969) and for triplets it is between 1.5 and 2.0 kg (Miettinen, 1954).

Twins weighing less than 1.8 kg contribute 68 per cent to the total perinatal loss and low birthweight affects both stillbirth and neonatal death rates. Although low birthweight is not an immediate cause of antepartum death, it may be a predisposing factor, and babies of less than 1.8 kg have more than five times the risk of being stillborn than those weighing more than 2.5 kg (Anderson, 1956). It seems likely that this increased mortality is due to those factors which cause intrauterine growth retardation (Bulmer, 1970), rather than low birthweight per se.

Neonatal mortality decreases with increasing birthweight to an optimum of about 3 kg, then above this weight mortality rises again. Under 2.5 kg neonatal loss is less in multiple births than in singletons (Bulmer, 1970) presumably because for a given weight multiple births are gestationally more advanced than singletons and are less likely to suffer from the problems of immaturity. On the other hand, deaths in the first year are higher for low birthweight twins than for singletons of the same weight (Alm, 1953).

Mean birthweight is lower and intra-pair weight differences greater when both twins die than when they both survive. Death may result from a competition effect due to, or merely reflected in, marked weight discrepancies (Parsons, 1964). When marked differences do occur, delivery of a large second twin becomes even more hazardous and is mainly responsible for the trebled incidence of fetal cerebral injury in twins, compared to singletons (Dunn, 1965).

Babies born to primigravidae have lower birthweights and five times as many primigravidae as multigravidae have babies of less than 1.0 kg (Spurway, 1962). Their babies also show greater weight discrepancies, which no doubt account in part for the higher mortality in this group, and also suggests that the intrauterine environment was less favourable (Parsons, 1964). Monoamniotic twins also have lower mean birthweights and a high incidence of intra-pair inequality, and they too have a poorer prognosis than other twins (Wharton, Edwards and Cameron, 1968). The same holds true for monochorionic twins, who are more retarded in growth than dichorionic twins and who also have a high mortality rate (Bulmer, 1970).

CAUSE OF DEATH

ABORTION

Multiple pregnancies often terminate in abortion. More than 40 per cent of all twin deaths occur before the 28th week and males are slightly more at risk than females. There is also a high late abortion loss in triplets. In Beacham and Beacham's series (1950) four of the 15 sets of triplets were lost at this time.

PREMATURITY

In all but the most recent literature the term prematurity does not differentiate between immature and small-for-dates babies, but simply groups together the heterogeneous group of low birthweight babies. All the same, if one excludes pregnancies which end in abortion, most multiple births die as a result of immaturity, low birthweight or causes associated with these conditions (Anderson, 1956; Barr and Stevenson, 1961; Butler and Alberman, 1969). About three-quarters of fetal and neonatal deaths are in low birthweight babies with no pathological lesion at post-mortem and such deaths occur with greater frequency than is found in singletons (Potter, 1963). Most of these babies are too small to survive but those between 2.0 and 2.5 kg do not die as a direct result of their weight but because of pathological conditions similar to those which lead to the deaths of larger babies (Anderson, 1956).

PERINATAL ASPHYXIA AND ANOXIA

Intrauterine anoxia occurs less frequently in twins than in singletons, but accounts for eight to ten per cent of their antepartum deaths and a slightly smaller percentage of their neonatal deaths (Barr and Stevenson, 1961; Potter, 1963; Myrianthopoulos, 1970). Intrauterine asphyxia is one of the main causes of death in low birthweight babies of more than 35 weeks' gestation (Dunn, 1965) but birth asphyxia is no more frequent than in singletons (Alm, 1953). MZ twins are twice as prone to anoxia as DZ twins, and boys are at greater risk than girls (Myrianthopoulos, 1970). Second-born infants are more likely to die from intrapartum causes not associated with birth trauma and babies dying in this way are significantly lighter than the surviving co-twin (Butler and Alberman, 1969).

BIRTH TRAUMA

Death due to trauma, with or without anoxia during labour, is four times more common in second-born twins and twice as common in first-born as it is in singletons. Twins dying from frank trauma are on average slightly heavier than the surviving co-twin. Girls are at greater risk than boys, despite the fact that boys are generally bigger than girls and one would expect them to suffer more from birth injury (Myrianthopoulos, 1970).

CONGENITAL MALFORMATION

A smaller proportion of twins die from malformation than do singletons (Butler and Alberman, 1969) and congenital malformation is not a major contributor to their overall mortality (Barr and Stevenson, 1961). This is because immaturity and low birthweight account for such a large percentage of the total deaths that other causes become relatively less significant. It is therefore more reasonable to make comparisons on the basis of death rates per thousand total births, when it becomes apparent that the incidence of lethal malformations is higher in twins, and even more common in those who are second-born (Dunn, 1965; Butler and Alberman, 1969). Twins seem to be particularly subject to the more severe abnormalities which result in a higher incidence of stillbirths than neonatal deaths (Anderson, 1956) especially in girls (Myrianthopoulos, 1970). Of the lethal malformations diagnosed in the first year of life the most common are circulatory, followed by anomalies of the central nervous system and the genitourinary system. The commonest single malformation is spina bifida (Barr and Stevenson, 1961).

RESPIRATORY DISTRESS

Respiratory difficulties in the newborn may be due to one of a multitude of causes, but are usually the result of hyaline membrane formation, pulmonary atelectasis or pneumonia. About 25 per cent of those who develop respiratory distress are twins, although the expected incidence is less than 10 per cent (Dunn, 1965). Atelectasis and pneumonia are more common causes of death in multiple births than in singletons (Barr and Stevenson, 1961) and deaths from hyaline membrane and pneumonia are four times higher in twins than in the general newborn population. This is a small difference when one considers that 50 per cent of twins weigh less than 2.5 kg (Potter, 1963). Second twins are twice as likely to die from hyaline membrane as their co-twins and about one-third of those affected by the disease are born at least 30 minutes after the first twin (Butler and Alberman, 1969). This suggests that the conditions which surround the birth of the second baby may pre-dispose to membrane formation and supports the hypothesis that it is associated with an increased incidence of pre-partum asphyxia (Potter, 1963; Butler and Alberman, 1969). Differences in zygosity and sex do not affect the incidence of respiratory difficulty (Myrianthopoulos, 1970) but con-cordance is more common in MZ than DZ pairs (Myrianthopoulos, Churchill and Baszynski, 1971). The length of pregnancy is a very important factor both in relation to incidence and to prognosis. Nearly all babies born between 28 and 35 weeks' gestation who die in the neonatal period suffer from hyaline membrane disease, but it is rarely the cause of death in those born nearer term (Dunn, 1965).

HAEMORRHAGE

Pulmonary and cerebral haemorrhage are common post-mortem findings in low birthweight babies, whether they are singleton or multiple births. Massive pulmonary haemorrhage is found particularly in small-for-dates babies and the smaller twin is at greater risk (Butler and Alberman, 1969). Intracranial haemorrhage may be due to birth trauma, asphyxia, or a combination of these. It is more common in immature than mature twins (Anderson, 1956) and the second twin is more at risk than the first (Butler and Alberman, 1969).

TWIN-TRANSFUSION SYNDROME

Injection studies in monochorial placentas often reveal large arterial or venous anastomoses on the fetal surface which seem to be of little functional importance (Davies et al, 1972). On the other hand, arteriovenous anastomoses are probably an important factor in the high mortality of mono-chorionic twins and many other intrauterine deaths are due to the twin-transfusion syndrome, in which vascular transplacental anastomoses are, in fact, inconspicuous.

It has been recognised for many years that occasionally twins of like sex have contrasting appearance at birth, one being pale and the other plethoric (Strong and Corney, 1967; Benirschke and Kim, 1973). Investigations show that the donor twin is anaemic and the recipient polycythaemic, with various additional aberrations of the blood picture, and it is presumed that one twin bleeds into the other. The situation has been clarified by the work of Naeye (1965) and Benirschke and Driscoll (1967) and there was a useful review of the problem by Rausen, Seki and Strauss in 1965. These authors, in addition to a comprehensive review of the literature, gave details of their own cases over a period of 10 years. They defined the twin-transfusion syndrome as a difference in haemoglobin concentration greater than 5 g per 100 ml, as they did not find a difference greater than this in DZ pairs, the highest difference in this group being 3.3 g per 100 ml. Similar observations were made by Abraham (1969). Criteria of this type can only be applied to liveborn babies and so Rausen and his colleagues also included as 'probable cases' those in which there were other signs known to be associated with the syndrome, such as hydramnios in one of the amniotic cavities or marked disparities in the size and weight of the twins, or of various organs, e.g. heart, liver or kidneys. With this approach it was estimated that of 130 monochorial twin pregnancies in their series 19 (15 per cent) warranted this diagnosis. These authors stressed that this was probably a conservative estimate since complete data were not available in every case. Most workers agree on this point, and those cases recognised at birth probably only form the tip of the iceberg, as many cases with minimal signs may not be detected and those more severely affected may have aborted.

It seems likely that we are observing a wide range of presentation resulting from various degrees of malfunction of the common circulation for which no single explanation is possible. Rausen, Seki and Strauss (1965) illustrate some of these points very well, particularly the lethal aspects of the situation. Of 38 twins with the transfusion syndrome, 25 died (66 per cent) and 12 of these weighed less than 500 g at delivery. Only four of the 19 affected pregnancies resulted in the survival of both twins. Amongst monochorial twins who did not survive, 34 per cent showed signs of the syndrome. In an earlier review of the literature, Smith and Benjamin (1968) found that about 15 per cent of all monochorial pregnancies are affected by the syndrome and 66 per cent of the babies die. It is rare for both babies to survive (Heinrichs, 1964) and the severe cases who do so are born with marked differences in weight, colour and haemoglobin levels, the plethoric recipient often being in a poorer state than the anaemic donor (Davies et al, 1972).

OTHER CAUSES

Other causes of death occur too infrequently for them to be numerically significant and in many infants, particularly macerated stillbirths, the cause of death is unknown. The most common maternal conditions associated with otherwise unexplained antepartum deaths are pre-eclampsia and antepartum haemorrhage. Prolapsed cord accounts for most of the intrapartum deaths, with early separation of the placenta and delay in delivering the second twin accounting for the remainder (Anderson, 1956).

MORBIDITY, DEVELOPMENT AND BEHAVIOUR

In general, multiple births behave in much the same way as singletons of the same weight and gestation, but a few conditions are more common, and others less frequent than one might expect. Twinning causes mental and physical defects perhaps due to intrauterine nutritional deprivation (Holley and Churchill, 1969) and on average these babies are smaller than expected. Gruenwald (1970) has shown that twins deviate from normal singleton growth standards early in the third trimester, their mean peak birthweight of 2.9 kg being reached at 39 weeks' gestation. Before 37 weeks, opposite-sex pairs conform to singleton standards and same-sex, monochorionic twins show the greatest deviation. After 37 weeks all twins fall below singleton levels. Monochorionic twins are often gestationally more immature than dichorionic pairs and in all instances they are at a greater disadvantage than other twins. Not only do they have a higher incidence of growth retardation, they also show more marked intra-pair weight discordance, suggesting that it is the monozygous (MZ) rather than the monochorial state which determines differences in growth and maturity patterns.

These differences in weight and maturity are important in determining not only the incidence and type of neonatal morbidity but also development and behaviour in infancy and childhood.

MORBIDITY

First week

Three of the more important causes of first week morbidity are hyaline membrane disease, hypoglycaemia and the twin-transfusion syndrome. Other conditions, such as malformation and rhesus haemolytic disease, present the same problem as in singletons, but may show discordance in multiple births.

Hyaline membrane disease. It has been mentioned already that hyaline membrane formation accounts for a large proportion of twin deaths, more so than in singletons. This difference cannot be accounted for purely on the basis of low birthweight and immaturity, since the frequency of the illness is out of all proportion to the incidence of these factors (Myrianthopoulos, Churchill and Baszynski, 1971), and it is related to birth order (Butler and Alberman, 1969), sex, and zygosity (Myrianthopoulos, Churchill and Baszynski, 1971).

Hypoglycaemia. Neonatal hypoglycaemia is common in all small-for-dates babies, and multiple pregnancy, with its extra demands on the mother's resources, is a frequent cause of intrauterine growth retardation. It is therefore not surprising that these infants are particularly prone to symptomatic hypoglycaemia. Reisner, Forbes and Cornblath (1965) have shown that there is no relationship with birth order or presentation, but the smaller baby has the higher risk of being affected. Boys are more likely to have pathologically low blood sugars than girls, especially if the co-twin is also male. Most of the affected babies are considerably underweight (at or below the tenth percentile) and marked intra-pair weight disparity is usual. Malnutrition is probably more to blame for this condition than overall growth retardation since many of these babies are below average for weight rather than for length. It is possible that neonatal hypoglycaemia is significant in the higher incidence of mental subnormality and slow development in the smaller baby.

Twin-transfusion syndrome. The twin-transfusion syndrome has been discussed in more detail in Chapters 3 and 13. Although it is usually the less severely affected infants who survive the perinatal period it is advisable to consider the possibility of this condition in all like-sex pairs who have markedly different birthweights, and at least check the haemoglobin levels as a screening measure at delivery.

Malformation. Multiple births have an increased risk of malformation, particularly the more severe varieties (Dunn, 1965), but there is little information in the literature concerning the incidence and mortality rates of specific abnormalities and most reports are concerned more with aetiology and inheritance. Monozygotic (MZ) twins are at greater risk of having some degree of abnormality especially if the placenta is monochorionic. Although concordance is more frequent in MZ than DZ pairs, discordance in identical twins is strikingly frequent (Fogel, Nitowsky and Gruenwald, 1965; Blake and Wreakes, 1972; Pembrey, 1972; Revesz, 1973) and also occurs in triplets (Tan et al, 1970b; Vestergaard, 1972).

Haemolytic disease. Rhesus haemolytic disease is no more common in multiple pregnancy than it is in singletons, but it presents more difficulties in antenatal management, with a consequent increase in mortality. The

outcome for each baby is not always the same, and in an analysis of 28 sets
of twins, Beischer, Pepperell and Barrie (1969) found that there were 10 pairs
where each twin had a different rhesus group, three pairs where both were
rhesus-negative and 15 pairs where both were rhesus-positive. The three
uniovular pairs were in this last group and all showed equal degrees of
haemolysis. There were seven pairs where the co-twins were affected differently, as judged by cord blood findings or clinical manifestations. In those
where the degree of anaemia differed, the smaller twin had the higher
haemoglobin. One pair in particular showed very marked differences in
severity but they also had different ABO blood groups, which no doubt
accounted for the fact that one died and the other survived.

Infancy and childhood

Cerebral palsy. There is a higher preponderance of twins amongst cases of
cerebral palsy than in the general population. Twins account for about 1.2
per cent of the total population yet they contribute between seven and nine
per cent to the cerebral palsy list (Bender, 1952; Greenspan and Deaver, 1953;
Yue, 1955). Many studies have suggested that twins are at high risk of
developing cerebral palsy and the smaller twin is particularly liable to be
afflicted (Asher and Schonell, 1950; Greenspan and Deaver, 1953; Illingworth
and Woods, 1960; Russell, 1961; Allen and Kallmann, 1962).

One of the best studies was made by Griffiths (1967) who analysed 78
twin pregnancies in which one or more members had cerebral palsy. There
were 58 normal co-twins, 82 cases of cerebral palsy and 16 stillbirths or
neonatal deaths. There was a higher than normal proportion (43 per cent)
of like-sex twins in the series and an even higher proportion (80 per cent)
among twin pairs with non-surviving co-twins. The incidence of immaturity
was 85 per cent, but this did not appear to be the only factor. There was a
difference in the probable cause of cerebral palsy as it affects first- and
second-born infants. The first-born twins were more often premature infants
presenting by the vertex and the commonest form of palsy was spastic
diplegia. Second-born twins were often mature and showed abnormalities
of presentation or symptoms of anoxia and usually presented with a more
severe type of palsy, often spastic tetraplegia or severe athetosis. It was
unusual for them to be diplegic. There were more normal survivors and
more neonatal deaths among second-born twins, and Griffiths suggested
that these differences in manifestation may help to throw further light on the
aetiology of cerebral palsy, especially of spastic diplegia, which appears to
be a separate condition rather than a milder form of spastic tetraplegia.

One possible factor in the aetiology of cerebral palsy in these cases might
be immaturity, as 56 out of 67 (73 per cent) of Griffith's cases occurred in
twins born before the 36th week of gestation. A second possibility is abnormalities of the present or previous pregnancies, but there is no evidence to
support this. Intra-pair differences do not seem to be involved either, but there
is a greater risk to those delivered by the breech and to second twins. In
other series (Russell, 1961; Eastman et al, 1962; Albermann, 1964) there

was also a slightly increased incidence of like-sex pairs compared with the expected incidence of 85 per cent and this suggests that there may be a higher proportion of monozygotic twins in a population of cerebral palsy children. The fact that there is discordance for all types of cerebral palsy in MZ pairs is strong evidence against a heredity factor. Allen and Kalman (1962) showed that whereas MZ twins were concordant for some forms of mental retardation there was no concordance when the retardation was associated with cerebral palsy and in 80 per cent of such cases there was a history of some kind of trauma.

Leukaemia. Many of the illnesses encountered by multiple births in their early years are the same and are just as common as those found in the general population, but twins under school age appear to have a lower incidence of leukaemia than other children (Jackson, Norris and Klauber, 1969). This may be due to selective elimination of twin zygotes in early embryonic life, as Hewitt and Stewart (1970) found that in children who died of malignant disease before they were 10 years old, there was a deficit of like-sex twins among the non-radiogenic cancers, which they felt might be due to the elimination of those whose neoplasms were the result of cell damage incurred at, or shortly after conception. Leukaemic twins and their unaffected siblings have greater birthweight disparities than the general twin population, and twin girls (especially if they are the heavier one of a pair) are at greater risk. More first- than second-born twins die of leukaemia but this is probably due to weight and sex differences rather than the result of birth order. Jackson, Norris and Klauber also found that it is unusual for MZ twins to be affected but when they are, the concordance rate is only 25 per cent. On the other hand Keith and Brown (1970) considered that most reported clinical cases occur in MZ twins and there is a high concordance rate in those presenting in the first year of life, but not later.

Triplets. In a follow up study of Finnish triplets, Miettinen and Grönroos (1965) found that all three members of the surviving MZ sets had remained well, apart from the usual childhood illnesses and none of them were found to have any abnormality. In only six sets containing identical twins was there concordance for a specific illness which did not affect the fraternal triplet. In the trizygotic sets only one triplet was affected in each case.

GROWTH AND DEVELOPMENT

Problems related to growth and development are the same as those found in all low birthweight infants (Alm, 1953; Wiener, 1962) though their difficulties may differ in degree. Low birthweight singletons tend to make up their deficiencies in weight and height by the time they are two years old unless their progress is hampered by recurrent illness or poor social conditions. By this age even the smallest of them is not much below the growth standard for mature controls, especially if they have remained well and had a good diet and satisfactory maternal care. But twins of less than 2.0 kg at birth, even when brought up under the most favourable conditions, never make up for their initial growth handicap (Drillien, 1958). Generally, small babies gain proportionately more weight than larger full-term infants, but twins put on less weight than singletons of the same size, especially if they weighed less than 2.5 kg at birth. At four years old, low birthweight infants, and twins in particular, are lighter and shorter than controls and they are also underweight for their height. The effects of maternal care, whether it be good or bad, can be recognised in all children, but the results of inadequate mothering are most marked in those who are small at birth, and in all twins regardless of their birthweight. Small-for-dates babies continue to be growth retarded in the pre-school years, to the extent that they have not caught up with babies of the same weight, but of shorter gestation (Drillien, 1961).

Little is known about the subsequent physical and mental development of triplets and quadruplets. According to Miettinen and Grönroos (1965), Finnish triplets surviving beyond three years old do not lag behind other children of the same age as far as physical development goes, and although the majority are of normal intelligence, three to four per cent are severely mentally handicapped (Miettinen, 1954).

INTELLIGENCE AND BEHAVIOUR

The mental and behavioural characteristics of twins have been studied in detail by many people, and although the results are contradictory on some points, there is little doubt that these children are handicapped in some way or another by their duality. Identical twins in particular are more vulnerable to the complications of pregnancy and delivery and hence to later neurological and psychological difficulties (Mittler, 1971).

Twins have an I.Q. eight points below that of singletons (Churchill and Henderson, 1974). They are often difficult to separate from each other and they tend to be less vocal and more introverted than singletons of the same age. The fact that they are small at birth is an important factor in retarding their intellectual and social development, making them more dependent and less well goal-orientated. They are not very good at following instructions and their interest in a particular task is often short-lived. Even allowing for low birthweight, by the time they are four years old they are still more dependent, less intense in their responses and have a lower I.Q. than singletons of the same age (Kranitz and Welcher, 1971).

Drillien (1959) has also shown that twins behave differently from singletons. Developmental quotients up to the age of two years fall steadily with decreasing birthweight and twins have lower scores than singletons. Low birthweight babies born to intelligent mothers show a steady improvement in developmental ability but no such improvement is found in those with mothers of poor intelligence. Small babies are slower in learning to walk and talk than fully grown controls and if they also come from a poor home their speech is generally more retarded than their locomotor development. On the whole, children born to primigravidae do better than those who come later in the family, especially if they were very small at birth or if the family background is far from ideal. Presumably this is because the mother has more time to devote to the babies. Surprisingly there is little evidence to show that the mental ability of those of the same birthweight is affected by the occurrence of cerebral symptoms in the neonatal period and it is possible that irritability, lethargy, apnoea, etc. in the first week is due more to cerebral immaturity than to cerebral injury.

Language and verbal reasoning

Unlike the low birthweight singleton whose reading ability is usually worse than his speech (Alm, 1953) language development in twins is inferior even when their non-verbal intelligence is normal, and by the time they are four years old their speech is six months behind that of singletons of the same age. Their language develops in the same way and at the same pace as in other children, but they start to talk later, despite the fact that they clearly understand what is said to them. Although identical twins have a higher incidence of birth complications they show no more speech impairment than fraternal twins, and in fact, unlike-sex pairs seem to do worst of all. Identical pairs, especially boys, often form a closed communications system and use their own secret language (cryptophasia) but this does not affect their verbal reasoning to any appreciable degree, although MZ twin boys may not say their first word until they are 18 months old (Mittler, 1970).

The association between social class and language, which is so important in singletons, does not seem to be so in twins. In fact, middle-class twins suffer relatively more than those from the working classes, possibly because they are less able to take advantage of their more favourable home background, whereas in the lowest social classes twins and singletons are equally adversely affected by their home conditions. Complications of pregnancy and delivery which affect the later development of most children do not affect twins to the same extent, and their intellectual and verbal behaviour seems to be governed more by postnatal than perinatal events (Mittler, 1970).

When they are older, twins have poorer verbal reasoning than singletons, though their results are better than triplets. Their lower scores in the eleven-plus examination are not explained by their gestational age, their place in the family or the age of their mother. The increased risks associated with mono-zygosity and birth order do not seem to be important either, and growth retardation is not a factor unless it is very marked. Twins brought up singly, e.g. because the other one died at birth, have scores only slightly below those of other children and they are much higher than the values obtained by those whose co-twin survived, despite the fact that many of the 'single' twins had considerably lower birthweights. These findings also support the view that prenatal complications and intrapartum difficulties have little or no effect on verbal reasoning in later childhood, but that retardation may be because twins maintain constant contact with each other, reducing their opportunities of communicating with adults and older children (Record, McKeown and Edwards, 1970; McKeown, 1970).

Although verbal scores do not correlate with birthweight, the smaller identical twin scores lower in the performance section of the I.Q. test than the larger baby (Churchill, 1967; McKeown, 1970; Babson and Phillips, 1973). By school age the heavier of like-sex twins has the highest I.Q., especially if the weight disparity at birth was more than 300 g. Unequal intrauterine conditions, with inadequate nutrition for brain development in the stunted child may be the reason for this later difference in ability (Willerman and Churchill, 1967; Kaelber and Pugh, 1969), but differences in weight do not seem to affect triplets in the same way (Miettinen and Grönroos, 1965).

Duality

Despite the many environmental factors which might contribute to the intellectual inferiority of twins, some people consider that it is inherent in twinning itself. Apart from their perinatal difficulties, there is a marked tendency for twins to be treated as a twosome, rather than as individuals, by their family and friends. Mittler (1971) describes a case of four-year-old twins who could not speak and whose I.Q.'s were reckoned to be in the low sixties. Mother was advised to stress their individuality, to dress them differently and not to refer to them collectively as 'the twins' but always to call them by name. A year later they were speaking fluently and their I.Q.s were 120.

OTHER PROBLEMS

Even when not treated as individuals, their mothers usually notice some differences between them. In the pre-school years these differences are mainly in temperament, irritability and crying, as well as in sleeping problems, toilet training and attention span. In twins whose birthweight differed by more than 700 g, the smaller twin (who was invariably small-for-dates) tends to have more problems. In twins of similar birthweight, behavioural differences are less noticeable and the smaller babies in this group tend to be immature at birth rather than growth-retarded. Birth sequence is not an important factor in behavioural differences (Matheny and Brown, 1971). At one year old, intra-pair differences are mainly in temperament and attention span, but by four years old the difference is mainly in sociability. The degree of sociability changes after the age of two and the older they get the greater the degree of individuality, but MZ twins remain more alike in their behaviour than DZ pairs (Wilson, Brown and Matheny, 1971).

CONCLUSION

Multiple births are at a disadvantage from the word 'go'. Their chance of survival depends not only on their number but also on many other factors, the most important of which are birthweight and gestational age. Those who do survive the neonatal period are liable to suffer some form of handicap, be it physical, mental or psychological, though in most cases their difficulties will be minimal and readily overcome.

References

Aaron, J. B., Silverman, S. H. & Halperin, J. (1961) Fetal survival in twin delivery. *American Journal of Obstetrics and Gynecology*, **81**, 331–334.

Abraham, J. M. (1969) Character of placentation in twins, as related to hemoglobin levels. *Clinical Pediatrics*, **8**, 526–530.

Abraham, R. C. (1958) *Dictionary of Modern Yoruba*. London: University of London Press.

Abrams, R. H. (1957) Double pregnancy. Report of a case with 35 days between deliveries. *Obstetrics and Gynecology*, **9**, 435–438.

Abroms, I. F., Bresnan, M. J. & Zuckerman, J. E. (1973) Cervical cord injuries secondary to hyperextension of the head in breech presentations. *Obstetrics and Gynecology*, **41**, 369–378.

Adams, D. L. & Fetterhoff, C. K. (1971) Locked twins. A case report. *Obstetrics and Gynecology*, **38**, 383–385.

Adeleye, J. A. (1972) Retained second twin in Ibadan: its fate and management. *American Journal of Obstetrics and Gynecology*, **114**, 204–207.

Aherne, W., Strong, S. J. & Corney, G. (1968) The structure of the placenta in the twin transfusion syndrome. *Biologia Neonatorum*, **12**, 121–135.

Aird, I. (1954) The conjoined twins of Kano. *British Medical Journal*, **i**, 831–837.

Aird, I. (1959) Conjoined twins—further observations. *British Medical Journal*, **i**, 1313–1315.

Albermann, E. D. (1964) Cerebral palsy in twins. *Guy's Hospital Report*, **113**, 285.

Albert, A., Randall, R. V., Smith, R. A. & Johnson, C. E. (1956) The Urinary Excretion of Gonadotrophin as a Function of Age. In *Hormones and the Aging Process* (Ed.) Engle, E. T. & Pincus, G. pp. 49–62. New York: Academic Press.

Alderman, B. A. (1973) Foetus acardius amorphus. *Postgraduate Medical Journal*, **49**, 102–105.

Allahbadia, N. K. (1962) Twin pregnancy associated with incompetence of the internal os. *British Medical Journal*, **i**, 1120.

Allegro, J. M. (1970) *The Sacred Mushroom and the Cross*. London: Hodder & Stoughton.

Allen, G. (1960) A differential method for estimation of type frequencies in triplets and quadruplets. *American Journal of Human Genetics*, **12**, 210–224.

Allen, G. (1965) Twin research: problems and prospects. *Progress in Medical Genetics*, **4**, 242–269.

Allen, G. & Firschein, I. L. (1957) The mathematical relations among plural births. *American Journal of Human Genetics*, **9**, 181–190.

Allen, G. & Kalman, F. J. (1962) Etiology of mental subnormality in twins. In *Expanding Goals of Genetics in Psychiatry* (Ed.) Kalman, F. J. London: Grune and Stratton.

Allen, G. & Schachter, J. (1971) Ease of conception in mothers of twins. *Social Biology*, **18**, 18–27.

Allen, J. P. (1972) Twin transfusion syndrome. *Northwest Medicine*, **71**, 296–298.

Alm, I. (1953) The longterm prognosis for prematurely born children. *Acta Paediatrica*, **42**, supplement **94**, 9–116.

Anderson, W. J. R. (1956) Stillbirth and neonatal mortality in twin pregnancy. *Journal of Obstetrics and Gynaecology of the British Empire*, **63**, 205–215.

Arey, L. B. (1922) Chorionic fusion and augmented twinning in the human tube. *Anatomical Record*, **23**, 253–262.

212

Asher, P. & Schonell, F. E. (1950) A survey of 400 cases of cerebral palsy in childhood. *Archives of Disease in Childhood*, **25**, 360.

Atlay, R. D. & Pennington, G. W. (1971) The use of clomiphene citrate and pituitary gonadotrophin in successive pregnancies: the Sheffield quadruplets. *American Journal of Obstetrics and Gynecology*, **109**, 402–407.

Babson, S. G. & Phillips, D. S. (1973) Growth and development of twins dissimilar in size at birth. *New England Journal of Medicine*, **289**, 937–940.

Ballantyne, J. W. (1902) *Manual of Antenatal Pathology and Hygiene*. Edinburgh: Green.

Banerjea, S. K. (1962) Index of placental function by endocrine assay and its clinical application in obstetric practice. *Journal of Obstetrics and Gynaecology of the British Commonwealth*, **69**, 963.

Barber-Riley, G., Goetzee, A. E., Richards, T. G. & Thomson, J. Y. (1961) The transfer of bromsulphthalein from the plasma to the bile in man. *Clinical Science*, **20**, 149–159.

Barlow, T. G. (1968) Congenital dislocation of the hip. *Hospital Medicine*, **2**, 571–577.

Barr, A. & Stevenson, A. C. (1961) Stillbirths and infant mortality in twins. *Annals of Human Genetics* (London), **25**, 131–140.

Barter, R. H., Hsu, I. & Erkenbeck, R. V. (1965) The prevention of prematurity in multiple pregnancy. *American Journal of Obstetrics and Gynecology*, **91**, 787–796.

Barter, R. H., Dusbabek, J. A., Tyndal, C. M. & Erkenbeck, R. V. (1963) Further experiences with the Shirodkar operation. *American Journal of Obstetrics and Gynecology*, **85**, 792–805.

Barton, R. F. (1946) The religion of the Ifugaos. No. 65 in *Titles in the Memoir Series of the American Anthropological Association. American Anthropologist*, New Series, **48**, No. 4, Part 2, 1–211.

Bascom, W. R. (1951) The Yoruba in Cuba. *Nigeria*, **37**, 14–20.

Basedow, H. (1925) *The Australian Aboriginal*. Adelaide: Preece.

Battaglia, F. C. & Lubchenko, L. O. (1967) A practical classification of newborn infants by weight and gestational age. *Journal of Pediatrics*, **71**, 159–163.

Baxter, R. H., Hsu, I., Erkenbeck, R. V. & Pugsley, L. Q. (1965) The prevention of prematurity in multiple pregnancy. *American Journal of Obstetrics and Gynecology*, **91**, 787–796.

Beacham, D. W. & Beacham, W. D. (1950) Triplet gestation and delivery with a report of fifteen cases. *Western Journal of Obstetrics and Gynecology* (Portland), **58**, 54–56.

Beazley, J. M. & Tindall, V. R. (1966) Changes in liver function during multiple pregnancy. *Journal of Obstetrics and Gynaecology of the British Commonwealth*, **73**, 658–661.

Beischer, N. A. & Fortune, D. W. (1968) Double monsters. *Obstetrics and Gynecology*, **32**, 158–170.

Beischer, N. A., Pepperell, R. J. & Barrie, J. U. (1969) Twin pregnancy and erythroblastosis. *Obstetrics and Gynecology*, **34**, 22–29.

Benda, C. E. (1952) *Developmental Disorders of Mentation and Cerebral Palsies*. New York: Grune and Stratton.

Bender, S. (1952) Twin pregnancy. A review of 472 cases. *Journal of Obstetrics and Gynaecology of the British Empire*, **59**, 510–517.

Benirschke, K. (1961) Accurate recording of twin placentation. A plea to the obstetrician. *Obstetrics and Gynecology*, **18**, 334–347.

Benirschke, K. (1970) Spontaneous chimerism in mammals. A critical review. *Current Topics in Pathology*, **51**, 1–61.

Benirschke, K. (1972a) Prenatal cardiovascular adaptation. In *Comparative Pathophysiology of Circulatory Disturbances; Advances in Experimental Medicine and Biology*, **22**, p. 3. (Ed.) Bloor, C. M. New York, London: Plenum Press.

Benirschke, K. (1972b) Origin and clinical significance of twinning. *Clinical Obstetrics and Gynecology*, **15**, 220–235.

Benirschke, K. & Driscoll, S. G. (1967) *The Pathology of the Human Placenta*. Berlin, Heidelberg, New York: Springer-Verlag.

Benirschke, K. & Kim, C. K. (1973) Multiple pregnancy. *New England Journal of Medicine*, **288**, 1276–1284, 1329–1336.

Bergsma, D. (Editor) (1967) Conjoined twins. *Birth Defects Original Article Series*, **3**(1). New York: National Foundation—March of Dimes.

Bernstine, R. L. & Borkowski, W. J. (1955) Prenatal fetal electrocardiography. *American Journal of Obstetrics and Gynecology*, **70**, 631–638.

Bertillon, M. (1874) Des combinaisons de sexe dans les grossesses gémellaires (doubles ou triples), de leur cause et de leur caractère ethnique. *Bulletin de la Société d'Anthropologie de Paris*, **9**, 267–290.

Bhargava, J., Chakravarty, A. & Raja, P. T. K. (1971) An anatomical study of the foetal blood vessels on the chorial surface of the human placenta. III Multiple pregnancies. *Acta Anatomica*, **80**, 465–479.

Bischoff, T. L. W. (1854) Quoted by Stockard, C. R. (1921). *American Journal of Anatomy*, **28**, 115–277.

Bishop, M. W. H. (1972) Genetically determined abnormalities of the reproductive system. *Journal of Reproduction and Fertility*, supplement **15**, 51–78.

Blake, G. B. & Wreakes, G. (1972) Clefts of the lip and palate in twins. *British Journal of Plastic Surgery*, **25**, 155–163.

Bleisch, V. R. (1964) Diagnosis of monochorionic twin placentation. *American Journal of Clinical Pathology*, **42**, 277–284.

Blondheim, S. H. (1947) The technique of foetal electrocardiography. *American Heart Journal*, **34**, 35–49.

Bolognesi, M. & Milani-Comparetti, M. (1970) Twinning and blood groups. I. ABO frequencies in twins and controls; immunological considerations. *Acta Geneticae Medicae et Gemellologiae*, **19**, 232–234.

Bonnevie, K. (1919) Om tvillingfödslers arvelig0hed. *Norsk Magazin for Laegevidenskaben*, **8**. (Cited in Dahlberg, G. (1923) Twins and Heredity. *Hereditas*, **4**, 27–32.)

Bourne, G. (1962) *The Human Amnion and Chorion*. London: Lloyd-Luke.

Bowes, W. A. & Droegemueller, W. (1968) Intrauterine transfusion of twins. *California Medicine*, **108**, 380–382.

Boyd, J. D. & Hamilton, W. J. (1970) *The Human Placenta*. Cambridge: Heffer.

British Perinatal Mortality Survey (1969) *Perinatal Problems—Second Report of the British Perinatal Mortality Survey*. Edinburgh, London: E. & S. Livingstone Ltd.

Broman, I. (1902) Ueber atypische Spermien (speciell beim Menschen) und ihre mögliche Bedeutung. *Anatomischer Anzeiger*, **21**, 497–531.

Brown, E. J. & Dixon, H. G. (1963) Twin pregnancy. *Journal of Obstetrics and Gynaecology of the British Commonwealth*, **70**, 251–257.

Brown, G. (1910) *Melanesians and Polynesians*. London: Macmillan.

Brown, R. T. K. & Vlaman, H. B. (1971) *Practical Neonatal Paediatrics*. Oxford, Edinburgh: Blackwell Scientific Publications.

Browne, F. J. (1946) *Antenatal and Postnatal Care*, 6th edition. London: Churchill.

Bruns, P. D. & Cooper, W. E. (1961) Basic factors influencing premature birth. *Clinical Obstetrics and Gynecology*, **4**, 341–351.

Bryan, E. M. (1975) Personal communication.

Bryan, E. M. & Kohler, H. G. (1974) The missing umbilical artery. I. Prospective study based on a maternity unit. *Archives of Disease in Childhood*, **49**, 844–851.

Bryan, E. & Slavin, B. (1974) Serum IgG levels in feto-fetal transfusion syndrome. *Archives of Disease in Childhood*, **49**, 908–910.

Bulmer, M. G. (1958) The numbers of human multiple births. *Annals of Human Genetics*, **22**, 158–164.

Bulmer, M. G. (1959a) Twinning rate in Europe during the war. *British Medical Journal*, i, 29–30.

Bulmer, M. G. (1959b) The effect of parental age, parity and duration of marriage on the twinning rate. *Annals of Human Genetics*, **23**, 454–458.

Bulmer, M. G. (1960) The twinning rate in Europe and Africa. *Annals of Human Genetics*, **24**, 121–125.

Bulmer, M. G. (1970) *The Biology of Twinning in Man*. Oxford: Clarendon Press.

Burnell, G. M. (1974) Maternal reaction to the loss of multiple births. A case of septuplets. *Archives of General Psychiatry*, **30**, 183–184.

Burrows, H. (1949) *Biological Actions of Sex Hormones*, 2nd edition. London: Cambridge University Press.

Butler, N. R. & Alberman, E. D. (1969) *Perinatal Problems—The Second Report of the 1958 British Perinatal Mortality Survey*. Edinburgh, London: E. & S. Livingstone Ltd.

Cameron, A. H. (1968) The Birmingham Twin Survey. *Proceedings of the Royal Society of Medicine*, **61**, 229–234.

Cameron, A. H., Robson, E. B., Wade-Evans, J. & Wingham, J. (1969) Septuplet conception: placental and zygosity studies. *Journal of Obstetrics and Gynaecology of the British Commonwealth*, **76**, 692–698.

Campbell, D. M. & MacGillivray, I. (1972) Comparison of maternal response in first and second pregnancies in relation to babyweight. *Journal of Obstetrics and Gynaecology of the British Commonwealth*, **79**, 684–693.

Campbell, D. M. & MacGillivray, I. (1975) The effect of a diet or a diuretic on the incidence of pre-eclampsia and babyweight. *British Journal of Obstetrics and Gynaecology*, in press.

Campbell, D. M., Campbell, A. J. & MacGillivray, I. (1975) Maternal characteristics of women having twin pregnancies. *Journal of Biosocial Science*, **6**, 463–470.

Campbell, D. M., Campbell, A. & MacGillivray, I. (1975) Blood pressure in twin pregnancy. In preparation.

Campbell, M. (1973) Incidence of cardiac malformations at birth and later, and neonatal mortality. *British Heart Journal*, **35**, 189–200.

Campbell, S. & Dewhurst, C. J. (1970) Quintuplet pregnancy diagnosed and assessed by compound ultrasound scanning. *Lancet*, **i**, 101.

Cannon, D. S. H. & Hartfield, V. J. (1964) Obstetrics in a developing country. A survey of 6 years' work in a Nigerian hospital. *Journal of Obstetrics and Gynaecology of the British Commonwealth*, **71**, 940–950.

Carter, C. O. (1965) The inheritance of common congenital malformations. *Progress in Medical Genetics*, **4**, 59.

Chamberlain, G. (1963) Hydatidiform mole in twin pregnancy. *American Journal of Obstetrics and Gynecology*, **87**, 140.

Chang, L. L. (1973) Storage of iron in fetal livers. *Acta Paediatrica Scandinavica*, **62**, 173–175.

Chappel, T. J. H. (1974) The Yoruba cult of twins in historical perspective. *Africa*, **44**, 250–265.

Christian, C. & Plummer, G. (1970) *God and One Redhead: Mary Slessor of Calabar*. London: Hodder & Stoughton.

Churchill, J. A. (1967) The relationship between intelligence and birthweight in twins. *Neurology*, **15**, 341–347.

Churchill, J. A. & Henderson, W. (1974) Perinatal factors affecting fetal development—twin pregnancy. *Birth Defects and Fetal Development*, Ch. 4 (Ed.) Mohhissi, K. S. Springfield, Illinois: Charles C. Thomas.

Compton, H. L. (1971) Conjoined twins. *Obstetrics and Gynecology*, **37**, 27.

Condie, R. (1974) *The Haemostatic Mechanism in Pregnancy with Particular Reference to Pre-eclampsia*. MD Thesis, University of Aberdeen.

Cook, R. C. M. (1971) Spina bifida and hydrocephalus. *British Medical Journal*, **iv**, 796–799.

Corner, G. W. (1955) The observed embryology of human single-ovum twins and other multiple births. *American Journal of Obstetrics and Gynecology*, **70**, 933–951.

Corney, G. & Aherne, W. (1965) The placental transfusion syndrome in monozygous twins. *Archives of Disease in Childhood*, **40**, 264.

Corney, G., Robson, E. B. & Strong, S. J. (1972) The effect of zygosity on the birth weight of twins. *Annals of Human Genetics*, **36**, 45–59.

Corston, J. McD. (1957) Twin survival. *Obstetrics and Gynecology*, **10**, 181.

Courey, N. G., Stull, R. L. & Fisher, B. (1970) Effect of bed rest upon urinary estriol excretion. *Obstetrics and Gynecology*, **178**, 35.

Cox, M. L. (1963) Incidence and aetiology of multiple births in Nigeria. *Journal of Obstetrics and Gynaecology of the British Commonwealth*, **70**, 878–884.

Crosby, W. M. & Gheen, D. L. Jr (1967) Intrauterine transfusion of twins; report of a case. *Obstetrics and Gynecology*, **29**, 674–676.

Cross, G. P., Hathaway, W. E. & McGaughey, H. R. (1973) Hyperviscosity in the neonate. *Journal of Pediatrics*, **82**, 1004–1012.

Csapo, A. I. (1961) The onset of labour. *Lancet*, **ii**, 2277.

Culley, P., Powell, J. & Waterhouse, J. (1970) Sequelae of neonatal jaundice. *British Medical Journal*, **iii**, 383–386.

Curtius, F. (1928)—quoted by Bulmer, M. G. in *The Biology of Twinning in Man (1970)*. Oxford: Clarendon Press.

Da Foe, A. R. (1934) The Dionne quintuplets. *Journal of the American Medical Association*, **103**, 673–677.

Dahlberg, G. (1926) *Twin Births and Twins from a Hereditary Point of View*. Stockholm: A. B. Tidens Tryckeri.

Dahlberg, G. (1952) Die Tendenz zu Zwillinsgeburten. *Acta Geneticae Medicae et Gemellologiae*, **1**, 80–88.

Danforth, C. H. (1916) Is twinning hereditary? *Journal of Heredity*, **7**, 195–202.

Danielson, C. (1960) Twin pregnancy and birth. *Acta Obstetrica et Gynecologia*, **39**, 63–87.

Davenport, C. B. (1920) Heredity of twin births. *Proceedings of the Society for Experimental Biology and Medicine*, **17**, 75–77.

Davenport, C. B. (1927) Does the male have an influence in human twin production? *Zeitschrift für induktive Abstammungs und Vererbungslehre*, **46**, 85–86.

Davies, P. A., Robinson, R. J., Scopes, J. W., Tizard, J. P. M. & Wigglesworth, J. S. (1972) *Medical Care of Newborn Babies; Clinics in Developmental Medicine No. 44/45*. Spastics International Medical Publications. London: William Heinemann Medical Books; Philadelphia: J. B. Lippincott.

Daw, E. & Walker, J. (1975) Biological aspects of twin pregnancy in Dundee. *British Journal of Obstetrics and Gynaecology*, **82**, 29–34.

De Angelis, R. R., Dursi, J. F. & Ibach, J. R. (1970) Successful separation of xiphopagus conjoined twins. *Annals of Surgery*, **172**, 302–305.

Deansley, R. (1966) The endocrinology of pregnancy and foetal life. In *Marshall's Physiology of Reproduction* (Ed.) Parkes, A. S. Vol. 3, p. 918. London: Longmans, Green.

DeCardi, C. N. (1899) Ju-Ju laws and customs in the Niger delta. *Journal of the Anthropological Institute of Great Britain and Ireland*, **29**, 51–64.

De George, F. V. (1970) Maternal and fetal disorders in pregnancies of mothers of twins. *American Journal of Obstetrics and Gynecology*, **108**, 975.

Dennerstein, G. J. (1971) Multiple pregnancy and cervical ligation with a case report of triplets. *Australian and New Zealand Journal of Obstetrics and Gynaecology*, **11**, 51–54.

Devereux, G. (1941) Mohave beliefs concerning twins. *American Anthropologist*, New Series, **43**, 573–592.

Devereux, G. (1960) *A Study of Abortion in Primitive Societies*. London: Yoseloff.

Diagnostic Indices in Pregnancy (1973) (Ed.) Hytten, F. E. & Lind, T. Basle: Documenta Geigy.

Donald, I. (1974) Sonar. What it can and cannot do in obstetrics. *Scottish Medical Journal*, **19**, 203–210.

Donaldson, R. S. & Kohl, S. G. (1965) Perinatal mortality in twins by sex. *American Journal of Public Health*, **55**, 1411–1418.

Donelly, M. (1956) The influence of multiple births on perinatal loss. *American Journal of Obstetrics and Gynecology*, **72**, 998.

Dorgan, L. T. & Clarke, P. E. (1956) Uterus didelphys with double pregnancy. *American Journal of Obstetrics and Gynecology*, **72**, 663–666.

Dornan, S. S. (1932) Some beliefs and ceremonies connected with the birth and death of twins among the South African natives. *South African Journal of Science*, **29**, 690–700.

Douglas, B. (1958) The role of environmental factors in congenital malformations. *Plastic and Reconstructive Surgery*, **22**, 94.

Drillien, C. M. (1958) A longitudinal study of the growth and development of prematurely and maturely born children. II. Physical development. *Archives of Disease in Childhood*, **33**, 423–431.

Drillien, C. M. (1959) A longitudinal study of the growth and development of prematurely and maturely born children. III Mental development. *Archives of Disease in Childhood*, **34**, 37–45.

Drillien, C. M. (1961) A longitudinal study of the growth and development of prematurely and maturely born children. VI Physical development in the age period 2 to 4 years. *Archives of Disease in Childhood*, **36**, 1–10.

Drucker, P., Finkel, J. & Savel, L. E. (1960) Sixty-five day interval between the births of twins. A case report. *American Journal of Obstetrics and Gynecology*, **80**, 761–763.

Duncan, J. M. (1865) On the comparative frequency of twin-bearing in different pregnancies. *Edinburgh Medical Journal*, **10**, 928–929.

Dunn, B. (1961) Bed rest in twin pregnancy. *Journal of Obstetrics and Gynaecology of the British Commonwealth*, **68**, 685–687.

Dunn, H. O., Lein, D. H. & Kenney, R. M. (1967) The cytological sex of a bovine anidian (amorphous) twin monster. *Cytogenetics*, **6**, 412–419.

Dunn, P. M. (1965) Some perinatal observations on twins. *Developmental Medicine and Child Neurology*, **7**, 121–134.

Eastman, N. J. (1961) Editorial comments. *Obstetrical and Gynaecological Survey*, **16**, 185.

Eastman, N. J., Kohl, S. G., Maisel, J. E. & Kavaler, F. (1962) The obstetrical background of 753 cases of cerebral palsy. *Obstetrical and Gynecological Survey*, **17**, 459.

Eckert, E. (1928) *Die Zwillings-geburten im Oberamt Tübingen aus den Jahren (1901–1925)*. Thesis, University of Tübingen.

Eckstein, H. B. (1968) Myelomeningocele, basic considerations. *Hospital Medicine*, **2**, 896–899.

Edmonds, H. W. (1954) The spiral twist of the normal umbilical cord in twins and in singletons. *American Journal of Obstetrics and Gynecology*, **67**, 102–120.

Edwards, J. H. (1968) The value of twins in genetic studies. *Proceedings of the Royal Society of Medicine*, **61**, 227–229.

Edwards, J. H., Cameron, A. H. & Wingham, J. (1967) *The Birmingham Twin Survey*. Cited in Strong, S. J. & Corney, G. (1967), p. 38.

Edwards, R. G. (1973) Physiological aspects of human ovulation, fertilization and cleavage. *Journal of Reproduction and Fertility*, supplement **18**, 87–101.

Ellis, A. B. (1894) *The Yoruba-speaking Peoples of the Slave Coast of West Africa*. London: Chapman & Hall.

Ellis, M. I., Coxon, A. & Noble, C. (1970) Intrauterine transfusion of twins. *British Medical Journal*, **i**, 609.

Epstein, F., Hochwald, G. M. & Ransohoff, J. (1973) Neonatal hydrocephalus treated by head wrapping. *Lancet*, **i**, 634–636.

Eriksson, A. W. (1964) Pituitary gonadotrophin and dizygotic twinning. *Lancet*, **ii**, 1298–1299.

Eriksson, A. W. & Fellman, J. (1967) Twinning in relation to the marital status of the mother. *Acta Genetica et Statistica Medica*, **17**, 385–398.

Evans-Pritchard, E. E. (1936) Customs and beliefs relating to twins among the Nilotic Nuer. *Uganda Journal*, **3**, 230–238.

Farrell, A. G. W. (1964) Twin pregnancy: a study of 1000 cases. *South African Journal of Obstetrics and Gynaecology*, **2**, 35–41.

Feldmann, H. U., Rupek, R. & Tenhaeff, D. (1971) Gehäuft mehrlingsschwangerschaften nach absetzen von ovulationshemmern? *Münchener Medizinische Wochenschrift*, **5**, 149–152.

Ferguson, W. F. (1964) Perinatal mortality in multiple gestations. A review of perinatal deaths from 1609 multiple gestations. *Obstetrics and Gynecology*, **23**, 854.

Ferm, V. H. (1969) Conjoined twinning in mammalian teratology. *Archives of Environmental Health*, **19**, 353–357.

Fisher, R. A. (1928) Triplet children in Great Britain and Ireland. *Proceedings of the Royal Society*, London, Series **B**, **102**, 286–311.

Fogel, B. J., Nitowsky, H. M. & Greenwold, P. (1965) Discordant abnormalities in monozygotic twins. *Journal of Pediatrics*, **66**, 64.

Ford, C. E. (1969) Mosaics and chimaeras. *British Medical Bulletin*, **25**, 104–109.

Fotheringham, J. (1974) Personal communication.

Francois, J., van Leuven, M. T. Matten & Vercanteren, M. (1972) Identical twins discordant for congenital spinal abnormality. *Acta Geneticae Medicae et Gemellologiae*, **21**, 107–115.

Frazer, J. G. (1900) *The Golden Bough. A Study in Magic and Religion*. 2nd edition, Vol. 1. London: Macmillan.

Frazer, J. G. (1905) *Lectures on the Early History of the Kingship*. London: Macmillan.

Frazier, E. F. (1942) The Negro family in Bahia, Brazil. *American Sociological Review*, **7**, 465–478.

Friedman, E. A. (1954) Graphic analysis of labour. *American Journal of Obstetrics and Gynecology*, **68**, 1568–1575.

Friedman, E. A. & Sachtleben, M. R. (1964) The effect of uterine overdistension on labor. I. Multiple pregnancy. *Obstetrics and Gynecology*, **23**, 164–172.

Fuchs, A. R. (1965) Role of oxytocin in the initiation of labour. *2nd International Congress of Endocrinology*, pp. 753–758. London: Excerpta Medica Congress Series, No. 82.

Fujikura, T. & Froehlich, L. A. (1971) Twin placentation and zygosity. *Obstetrics and Gynecology*, **37**, 34–43.

Fullerton, W. T., Hytten, F. E., Klopper, A. & McKay, E. (1965) A case of quadruplet pregnancy. *Journal of Obstetrics and Gynaecology of the British Commonwealth*, **72**, 791–796.

Gaehtgens, G. (1936) Klinischer Beitrag zur Pathogenese des akuten Hydramnions. *Monatsschrift für Geburtschilfe und Gynäkologie*, **103**, 40–48.

Garrett, W. J. (1960) Uterine overdistension and the duration of labour. *Medical Journal of Australia*, **47**, 376.

Gedda, L. (1951) *Studio dei Gemelli*. Rome: Edizioni Orizzonte Medico.

Gedda, L. (1961) *Twins in History and Science*. Springfield, Illinois: Thomas.

Gedda, L., Segni, G., Andreani, D., Casa, D. & Di Marco, G. (1969) Diabetes and gemellogenesis. *Acta Geneticae Medicae et Gemellologiae*, **19**, 87–90.

Gellman, V. (1959) Congenital hydrocephalus in monovular twins. *Archives of Disease in Childhood*, **34**, 274.

Gemme, G. & Verri, B. (1968) Aspetti clinici e biologici neonatali legati a trasfusione materno-fetale, feto-fetale e feto-materna. *Minerva Nipiologica*, **18**, 113–115.

Gemzell, C. & Roos, P. (1966) Pregnancies following treatment with human gonadotrophins, with special reference to the problem of multiple births. *American Journal of Obstetrics and Gynecology*, **94**, 490–496.

Gemzell, C. A., Roos, P. & Loeffler, F. E. (1968) Follicle-stimulating hormone extracted from the human pituitary. In *Progress in Infertility* (Ed.) Behrman, S. J. & Kistner, R. W. p. 375. London: Churchill.

Giblett, E. R. (1969) *Genetic Markers in Human Blood*. Oxford, Edinburgh: Blackwell Scientific Publications.

Giles, P. (1908) Abandonment and exposure. In *Encyclopaedia of Religion and Ethics* (Ed.) Hastings, J. Vol. 1, p. 3. Edinburgh: Clark.

Gillim, D. L. & Hendricks, C. H. (1953) Holocardius: a review of the literature and case report. *Obstetrics and Gynecology*, **2**, 647.

Gittlesohn, A. & Milham, S. (1964) Statistical study of twins. *American Journal of Public Health*, **54**, 286.

Graves, L. R. Jr, Adams, J. Q. & Schreier, P. C. (1962) The fate of the second twin. *Obstetrics and Gynecology*, **19**, 246–250.

Green, J. W. & Touchstone, J. C. (1963) Urinary estriol as an index of placental function. *American Journal of Obstetrics and Gynecology*, **85**, 1.

Green, M. & Behrendt, H. (1973) Sweating responses of neonates to local thermal stimulation. *American Journal of Diseases of Children*, **125**, 20–25.

Greenhill, J. P. (1955) *Obstetrics*, 11th edition. Philadelphia: Saunders.

Greenspan, L. & Deaver, G. G. (1953) Clinical approach to the etiology of cerebral palsy. *Archives of Physical Medicine and Rehabilitation*, **34**, 478.

Greulich, W. W. (1930) The incidence of human multiple births. *American Naturalist*, **64**, 142–153.

Greulich, W. W. (1934) Heredity in human twinning. *American Journal of Physical Anthropology*, **19**, 391–431.

Griffiths, M. (1967) Cerebral palsy in multiple pregnancy. *Developmental Medicine and Child Neurology*, **9**, 173.

Gruenwald, P. (1970) Environmental influences on twins apparent at birth. A preliminary study. *Biology of the Neonate*, **15**, 79–93.

Guttmacher, A. F. (1937) An analysis of 521 cases of twin pregnancy. *American Journal of Obstetrics and Gynecology*, **34**, 76–84.

Guttmacher, A. F. (1939a) An analysis of 573 cases of twin pregnancy. *American Journal of Obstetrics and Gynecology*, **38**, 277–288.

Guttmacher, A. F. (1939b) Clinical aspects of twin pregnancy. *Medical Clinics of North America*, **23**, 427–447.

Guttmacher, A. F. & Kohl, S. G. (1958) The fetus of multiple gestations. *Obstetrics and Gynecology*, **12**, 528–541.

Hack, M., Brish, M., Serr, D. M., Insler, V. & Lunenfeld, B. (1970) Outcome of pregnancy after induced ovulation: follow-up of pregnancies and children born after gonadotrophin therapy. *Journal of the American Medical Association*, **211**, 791–797.

Hack, M., Brish, M., Serr, D. M., Insler, V., Salomy, M. & Lunenfeld, B. (1972) Outcome of pregnancy after induced ovulation: follow-up of pregnancies and children born after clomiphene therapy. *Journal of the American Medical Association*, **220**, 1329–1333.

Halbert, D. R. & Christakos, A. C. (1970) Discordance of sexual anomalies in monozygotic twins. *Obstetrics and Gynecology*, **36**, 388.

Hall, M. (1970) *Assessment of the Effects of Folic Acid Deficiency in Pregnancy*. MD Thesis, Aberdeen University.

Hambly, W. D. (1937) *Source Book for African Anthropology*, Part II. *Anthropological Series*, Vol. 26. Chicago: Field Museum of Natural History.

Hamilton, W. J. (1954) A note on the embryology of twinning. *Proceedings of the Royal Society of Medicine*, **47**, 682–683.

Hamilton, W. J. & Poswillo, D. E. (1972) Placenta of marmosets. *Journal of Anatomy*, **111**, 505.

Hamilton, W. J., Brown, D. & Spiers, B. G. (1959) Another case of quadruplets. *Journal of Obstetrics and Gynaecology of the British Empire*, **66**, 409–412.

Hamlett, G. W. D. (1933) Observations on the embryology of the badger. *Anatomical Record*, **53**, 283–303.

Hammond, J. (1952) Fertility. In *Marshall's Physiology of Reproduction*, 3rd edition, Vol. 2 (Ed.) Parkes, A. S. London: Longmans.

Hanart, E. & Kalin, A. (1972) Hereditary and empirical prognosis of inheritance in cleft lip, maxilla and palate, based on 326 cases, among 309 non-selected Swiss families. *Journal de Génétique Humaine* (Geneva), **20**, 93–134.

Hanson, L. A. & Winberg, J. (1972) Breast milk and defence against infection in the newborn. *Archives of Disease in Childhood*, **47**, 845–848.

Harris, J. R. (1913) *Boanerges*. Cambridge: University Press.

Harris, J. R. (1922) A recent twin murder in South Africa. *Folklore*, **33**, 214–223.

Harris, R. (1928) *The Piety of the Heavenly Twins* (Woodbrooke Essays No. 14). Cambridge: Heffer.

Harrison, K. A. (1969) Changes in blood volume produced by treatment of severe anaemia in pregnancy. *Clinical Science*, **36**, 197–207.

Hartland, E. S. (1921) Twins. In *Encyclopaedia of Religion and Ethics* (Ed.) Hastings, J. Vol. 12, p. 491. Edinburgh: Clark.

Hay, S. & Wehrung, D. A. (1970) Congenital malformations in twins. *American Journal of Human Genetics*, **22**, 662.

Heinrichs, E. H. (1964) The intra-uterine feto-fetal transfusion. Pathophysiology of a syndrome. *Journal of the American Medical Association*, **187**, 862–864.

Hellin, D. (1895) *Die Ursache der Multiparität der Unipaaren Tiere Überhaupt und der Zwillingsschwangerschaft beim Menschen insbesondere.*

Hendricks, C. H. (1966) Twinning in relation to birth weight, mortality, and congenital anomalies. *Obstetrics and Gynecology*, **27**, 47.

Herlitz, G. (1941) Zur Kenntnis der anämischen und polyzytämischen zustände bei Neugeborenen, sowie des Icterus gravis neonatorum. *Acta Paediatrica* (Uppsala), **29**, 211–253.

Herrlin, K. M. & Hauge, M. (1967) The determination of triplet zygosity. *Acta Genetica et Statistica Medica*, **17**, 81–95.

Herskovits, M. J. (1938) *Dahomey: An Ancient West African Kingdom*, Vol. 1. New York: Augustin.

Hertig, A. T. (1967) The overall problem in man. In *Comparative Aspects of Reproductive Failure* (Ed.) Benirschke, K. p. 11. Berlin, Heidelberg, New York: Springer-Verlag.

Heuser, R. L. (1967) Multiple births, United States—1964. *Vital and Health Statistics*, **21**(14), 1–50.

Hewitt, D. & Stewart, A. (1970) Relevance of twin data to intrauterine selection. *Acta Geneticae Medicae et Gemellologiae*, **19**, 83–86.

Hirst, J. C. (1939) Maternal and fetal expectations with multiple pregnancy. *American Journal of Obstetrics and Gynecology*, **37**, 634–643.

Hollander, H-J. (1969) Monoamniotische Zwillinge. *Zeitschrift für Gebürtshilfe und Gynäkologie*, **171**, 292–300.

Holley, W. L. & Churchill, J. A. (1969) *Physical and Mental Deficits of Twinning. Perinatal Factors Affecting Human Development.* P.A.H.O. publications, No. 185. Washington: Pan American Health Organisation.

Holt, S. B. (1968) *The Genetics of Dermal Ridges.* Springfield, Illinois: Thomas.

Hon, E. H. & Hess, O. W. (1960) The clinical value of fetal electrocardiography. *American Journal of Obstetrics and Gynecology*, **79**, 1012–1023.

Hose, C. & McDougall, W. (1912) *The Pagan Tribes of Borneo.* London: Macmillan.

Hueter, C. C. (1845) *Der Einfache Mutterkuchen der Zwillinge.*

Human Genetics (1972) Prepared by the Standing Medical Advisory Committee for the Central Health Services Council, the Secretary of State for Social Services and the Secretary of State for Wales. London: Department of Health and Social Security.

Hyrtl, J. (1870) *Die Blutgefässe der Menschlichen Nachgeburt.* Vienna: Braumüller.

Hytten, F. E. & Leitch, I. (1964) *The Physiology of Human Pregnancy.* Oxford: Blackwell.

Hytten, F. E. & Lind, T. (1973) *Diagnostic Indices in Pregnancy.* Basle: Documenta Geigy.

Idelberger, K. (1929) Die Zwillings pathologie des angeborenen Klumpfuss. Beilagehaft zur. *Zeitschrift für Ornithologie und praktishe Geflügelzucht*, **69**.

Idelberger, K. (1951) *Der Erb pathologie der segamaunter angeborenen Heift Vervenkung.* Munchen, Berlin: Urban und Schwarzenberg.

Idowu, E. B. (1962) *Olódùmarè: God in Yoruba Belief.* London: Longmans Green.

Illingworth, R. S. & Woods, G. E. (1960) The incidence of twins in cerebral palsy and mental retardation. *Archives of Disease in Childhood*, **35**, 333.

Ingalls, T. H. & Bazemore, M. K. (1969) Prenatal events antedating the birth of thoracopagus twins. *Archives of Environmental Health*, **19**, 358–364.

Ingalls, T. H., Philbrook, R. & Majima, A. (1969) Conjoined twins in zebra fish. *Archives of Environmental Health*, **19**, 344–352.

Jackson, E. W., Norris, F. D. & Klauber, M. R. (1969) Childhood leukaemia in California-born twins. *Cancer*, **23**, 913–919.

Jacobson, A., Marshall, J. R., Ross, G. T. & Cargille, C. M. (1968) Clomiphene and plasma gonadotrophins. *Lancet*, **i**, 1371.

James, W. H. (1972) Secular changes in dizygotic twinning rates. *Journal of Biosocial Science*, **4**, 427–434.

Javert, C. T. (1957) *Spontaneous and Habitual Abortion.* New York: Blakiston.

Jeanneret, O. & MacMahon, B. (1962) Secular changes in rates of multiple births in the United States. *American Journal of Human Genetics*, **14**, 410–425.

Jeffcott, L. B. & Whitwell, K. E. (1973) Twinning as a cause of foetal and neonatal loss in the thoroughbred mare. *Journal of Comparative Pathology*, **83**, 91–106.

Jeffrey, R. L., Bowes, W. A. & Delaney, J. J. (1974) Role of bed rest in twin pregnancy. *Obstetrics and Gynecology*, **43**, 822–826.

Jeffreys, M. D. W. (1953) Twin births among Africans. *South African Journal of Science*, **50**, 89–93.

Jeffreys, M. D. W. (1963) The cult of twins among some African tribes. *South African Journal of Science*, **59**, 97–107.

Jenkins, R. L. (1927) Twin and triplet birth ratios: the inter-relations of the frequencies of plural births. *Journal of Heredity*, **18**, 387–394.

Jewelwicz, R., James, S. L., Finster, M., Dyrenfurth, J., Warren, M.P. & Wiele, R. L. V. (1972) Quintuplet gestation after ovulation induction with menopausal gonadotrophins and pituitary luteinising hormone. *Obstetrics and Gynecology*, **40**, 1–5.

Johnstone, F. & MacGillivray, I. (1975) Relationship between protein intake and nitrogen output in pregnancy. In preparation.

Jonas, E. G. (1963) The value of prenatal bed-rest in multiple pregnancy. *Journal of Obstetrics and Gynaecology of the British Commonwealth*, **70**, 461–464.

Jost, A. (1970) Hormonal factors in the sex differentiation of the mammalian foetus. *Philosophical Transactions of the Royal Society*, Series B, **259**, 119–131.

Jost, A. (1974) Mechanisms of normal and abnormal sex differentiation in the fetus. In *Birth Defects and Fetal Development: Endocrine and Metabolic Factors* (Ed.) Moghissi, K. S. p. 116. Springfield, Illinois: Thomas.

Junod, H. A. (1927) *The Life of a South African Tribe*, 2nd edition. Vol. II. *Mental Life*. London: Macmillan.

Kaelber, C. T. & Pugh, T. F. (1969) Influence of intrauterine relations on the intelligence of twins. *New England Journal of Medicine*, **280**, 1030–1034.

Kaestner, S. (1912) *The Development of Double Formation of Man and the Higher Vertebrates. A Collection of Anatomical and Physical Lectures and Essays by Gaup and Trendelenburg*, 2. Jena.

Kandror, I. S. (1961) Physical development of newborn infants and children up to 3 years (born in the Arctic). *Pediatriya*, **40** (6), 41–42.

Kang, Y. S. & Cho, W. K. (1962) The sex ratio at birth and other attributes of the newborn from maternity hospitals in Korea. *Human Biology*, **34**, 38–48.

Karn, M. N. (1952) Birthweight and length of gestation in twins together with maternal age, parity and survival rate. *Annals of Eugenics*, **16**, 365–377.

Karn, M. (1953) Twin data: a further study of birthweight, gestational time, maternal age, order of birth and survival. *Annals of Eugenics*, **17**, 233–248.

Keay, A. J. (1958) The significance of twins in mongolism in the light of new evidence. *Journal of Mental Deficiency Research*, **2**, 1.

Keith, L. & Brown, E. (1970) Leukaemia in twins. *Acta Geneticae Medicae et Gemellologiae* (Roma), **19**, 83–86.

Keith, L., Cestaro, A. & Elias, I. (1967) Fetus holoacardius: a complication of monochorial twinning. *Chicago Medical School Quarterly*, **27**, 30–35.

Kemsley, W. F. F., Billewicz, W. Z. & Thomson, A. M. (1962) A new weight-for-height standard based on British anthropometric data. *British Journal of Preventive and Social Medicine*, **16**, 189–195.

Kennedy, J. F. & Donahue, R. P. (1969) Binucleate human oocytes from large follicles. *Lancet*, **i**, 754–755.

Kerr, M. G. & Rashad, M. N. (1966) Autosomal trisomy in a discordant monozygotic twin. *Nature*, **212**, 726–727.

Keys, A., Brožek, J., Henschel, A., Mickelsen, O. & Taylor, H. L. (1950) *The Biology of Human Starvation*. University of Minnesota Press, Minneapolis.

Khanna, K. K., Roy, P. B. & Bhatt, V. P. (1969) Female pseudo-hermaphroditism in conjoined twins. *Indian Journal of Medical Science*, **23**, 201–205.

Khunda, S. (1972) Locked twins. *Obstetrics and Gynecology*, **39**, 453–459.

Kimball, A. P. & Rand, P. R. (1950) A maneuver for the simultaneous delivery of chin-to-chin locked twins. *American Journal of Obstetrics and Gynecology*, **59**, 1167.

Kindred, J. E. (1944) Twin pregnancies with one twin blighted. *American Journal of Obstetrics and Gynecology*, **48**, 642.

Klebe, J. G. & Ingomar, C. J. (1972) The fetoplacental circulation during parturition illustrated by the inter-fetal transfusion syndrome. *Pediatrics*, **49**, 112–116.

Klein, J. (1964) Perinatal mortality in twin pregnancy. *Obstetrics and Gynecology*, **23**, 738–744.

Kloosterman, G. J. (1963) The "third circulation" in identical twins. *Nederlands Tijdschrift voor Verloskunde en Gynaecologie*, **63**, 395–412.

Knox, G. & Morley, D. (1960) Twinning in Yoruba women. *Journal of Obstetrics and Gynaecology of the British Commonwealth*, **67**, 981–984.

Koivisto, M., Sequeiros, M. & Kranse, U. (1972) Neonatal symptomatic hypoglycaemia: a follow up study of 151 children. *Developmental Medicine and Child Neurology*, **14**, 603–614.

Komai, T. & Fukuoka, G. (1936) Frequency of multiple births among the Japanese and related peoples. *American Journal of Physical Anthropology*, **21**, 433–447.

Kranitz, M. A. & Welcher, D. W. (1971) Behavioural characteristics of twins. *Johns Hopkins Medical Journal*, **129**, 1–5.

Kurtz, G. R., Davis, L. L. & Loftus, J. B. (1958) Factors influencing the survival of triplets. *Obstetrics and Gynecology*, **12**, 504–508.

Lachelin, G. C. L., Brant, H. A., Swyer, G. I. M., Little, V. & Reynolds, E. O. R. (1972) Sextuplet pregnancy. *British Medical Journal*, **i**, 787–790.

Lagercrantz, S. (1941) Über willkommene und unwillkommene zwillinge in Afrika. *Etnologiska Studier*, **12–13**, 5–292.

Lamy, M., Frézal, J., Grouchy, J. de & Chryssostomidou, M. (1955) L'age maternel et le rang de naissance dans un echantillon de jumeaux. *Acta Genetica et Statistica Medica*, Basle, **5**, 403–419.

Landes, R. (1940) Fetish worship in Brazil. *Journal of American Folklore*, **53**, 261–271.

Larson, S. L. & Banner, E. A. (1966) Hydrocephalus. A 30 year study. *Obstetrics and Gynecology*, **28**, 571.

Larson, S. L., Wilson, R. B. & Titus, J. L. (1969) Monoamniotic hydrocephalic twins with survival. *Obstetrics and Gynecology*, **34**, 1969.

Law, R. G. (1967) *Standards of Obstetric Care: the Report of the North West Metropolitan Regional Obstetric Survey*. Edinburgh: E. & S. Livingstone.

Lawrence, R. F. (1949) Locked twins. *Journal of Obstetrics and Gynaecology of the British Commonwealth*, **56**, 58.

Lawson, J. B. (1961) Pre-eclampsia and eclampsia in Nigeria. *Pathologia et Microbiologia*, **24**, 478–483.

Leach, M. (Ed.) (1949) Dioscuri. In *Standard Dictionary of Folklore, Mythology and Legend*, Vol. 1, p. 314. New York: Funk & Wagnalls.

Leading Article (1968) *British Medical Journal*, **i**, 534.

Leading Article (1970) *British Medical Journal*, **iii**, 657–658.

Lees, M. M., Scott, D. B. & Kerr, M. G. (1970) Haemodynamic changes associated with labour. *Journal of Obstetrics and Gynaecology of the British Commonwealth*, **77**, 29–36.

Lenz, F. (1933) Zur Frage der Ursachen von Zwillingsgeburten. *Archiv für Rassen und Gesellschaftsbiologie*, **27**, 294–318.

Lenz, F. (1934) In *Human Heredity* (Ed.) Bauer, E., Fischer, E. & Lenz, F. London: Allen and Unwin.

Leonard, A. G. (1906) *The Lower Niger and its Tribes*. London: Macmillan.

Letchworth, A. T., Howard, L. & Chard, T. (1974) Placental lactogen levels during bed rest. *Obstetrics and Gynecology*, **43**, 702–703.

Liggins, G. C., Kennedy, P. C. & Holm, L. W. (1967) Failure of initiation of parturition after electrocoagulation of the pituitary of the fetal lamb. *American Journal of Obstetrics and Gynecology*, **98**, 1080.

Little, W. A. & Friedman, E. A. (1958) The twin delivery—factors influencing second twin survival. *Obstetrical and Gynecological Survey*, **13**, 611–623.

Loeb, E. M. (1958) The twin cult in the Old and the New World. *Miscellanea Paul Rivet Octogenario Dicata*, pp. 151–174. *XXXI Congreso Internacional De Americanistas Universidad Nacional Autónoma De México*.

Loeb, J. (1909) Ueber die chemischen Bedingungen für die Entstehung eineiiger Zwillinge beim Seeigel. *Archiv für Entwicklungsmechanik der Organismen*, **27**, 119–140.

Long, E. C. (1963) The placenta in lore and legend. *Bulletin of the Medical Library Association*, **51**, 233–241.

Loraine, J. A. (1963) Some clinical applications of assays of pituitary gonadotrophins in human urine. In *Pituitary–ovarian Endocrinology* (Ed.) Dorfman, R. I. & Neves e Castro, M. pp. 183–196. San Francisco: Holden-Day.

Lorber, J. (1972a) Congenital malformations of the central nervous system. *British Journal of Hospital Medicine*, **8**, 37–48.

Lorber, J. (1972b) Spina bifida cystica: results of treatment of 270 consecutive cases with criteria for selection for the future. *Archives of Disease in Childhood*, **47**, 854–872.

Lorber, J. (1972c) The use of isosorbide in the treatment of hydrocephalus. *Developmental Medicine and Child Neurology* (London), **14**, supplement 27, 87–93.

Lugo, G. & Cassady, G. (1971) Intrauterine growth retardation. *American Journal of Obstetrics and Gynecology*, **109**, 615–622.

McArthur, J. W. (1942) Relations of body size to litter size and to the incidence of fraternal twins. *Journal of Heredity*, **33**, 87–91.

McArthur, N. R. (1949) *A Statistical Study of Human Twin Genetics*. Ph.D. Thesis, University of London.

McArthur, N. (1952) A statistical study of human twinning. *Annals of Eugenics*, **16**, 338–350.

McClure, H. I. (1937) Multiple pregnancy. *Ulster Medical Journal*, **6**, 284–292.

MacDonald, A. D. (1964) Mongolism in twins. *Journal of Medical Genetics*, **1**, 39.

MacDonald, I. A. (1957) Suture of the cervix for inevitable miscarriage. *Journal of Obstetrics and Gynaecology of the British Empire*, **64**, 346–350.

MacDonald, R. R. (1962) Management of second twin. *British Medical Journal*, **i**, 518–522.

McFee, J. G., Lord, E. L., Jeffrey, R. L., O'Meara, O. P., Josepher, H. J., Butterfield, L. J. & Thompson, H. E. (1974) Multiple gestations in high fetal number. *Obstetrics and Gynecology*, **44**, 99–106.

MacGillivray, I. (1958) Some observations on the incidence of pre-eclampsia. *Journal of Obstetrics and Gynaecology of the British Empire*, **65**, 536–539.

MacGillivray, I. (1961) Hypertension in pregnancy and its consequences. *Journal of Obstetrics and Gynaecology of the British Commonwealth*, **68**, 557–569.

MacGillivray, I. (1970) The changing incidence of twinning in Scotland in 1939–1968. *Acta Geneticae Medicae et Gemellologiae*, **19**, 26–29.

MacGillivray, I. & Campbell, D. M. (1975) Physiological changes in twin pregnancy. In preparation.

MacGillivray, I., Campbell, D. M. & Duffus, G. M. (1971) Maternal metabolic response to twin pregnancy in primigravidae. *Journal of Obstetrics and Gynaecology of the British Commonwealth*, **78**, 530.

MacGillivray, I., Rose, G. A. & Rowe, B. (1969) Blood pressure survey in pregnancy. *Clinical Science*, **37**, 395–407.

McGowan, G. W. (1970) Cervical incompetence in multiple pregnancy. *Obstetrics and Gynecology*, **35**, 589–591.

McKeown, T. (1970) Prenatal and early postnatal influences on measured intelligence. *British Medical Journal*, **iii**, 63–67.

McKeown, T. & Record, R. G. (1952) Observations on foetal growth in multiple pregnancy in man. *Journal of Endocrinology*, **8**, 386–401.

McKeown, T. & Record, R. G. (1960) Malformations in a population observed for five years after birth. In *CIBA Foundation Symposium on Congenital Malformations, April, 1967* (Ed.) G. E. W. Wolstenholme and C. M. O'Connor. pp. 2–21.

MacMillan, D. R., Brown, A. M., Mathany, A. P. & Wilson, J. (1973) Relations between placental concentrations of chorionic somatomammotrophin (placental lactogen) and growth: A study using the twin method. *Pediatric Research*, **7**, 719–723.

Mall, F. P. (1908) Quoted by Stockard, C. R. (1921) *American Journal of Anatomy*, **28**, 115–277.

Masson, G. M. (1974) *Studies of Plasma Oestriol Concentration during Human Pregnancy*. MD Thesis, Aberdeen University.

Matheny, A. P. Jr & Brown, A. M. (1971) The behaviour of twins: effects of birthweight and birth sequence. *Child Development*, **42**, 251–257.

Matsunaga, E. (1966) Some remarks on the biology of twins. *Japanese Journal of Human Genetics*, **11**, 227–228.

Mawdsley, T., Rickman, P. P. & Roberts, J. R. (1967) Long term results of early operation of open myelomeningoceles and encephaloceles. *British Medical Journal*, **i**, 663–666.

Mayer, C. F. (1952a) Sextuplets and higher multiparous births. Part 1. Multiparity and sextuplets. *Acta Geneticae Medicae et Gemellologiae*, **1**, 118–135.

Mayer, C. F. (1952b) Sextuplets and higher multiparous births. Part 2. Septuplets and higher births. *Acta Geneticae Medicae et Gemellologiae*, **1**, 242–275.

Mayr, W. R., Pausch, V. & Mickerts, D. (1969) Serological findings on quadrizygotic quadruplets. *Vox Sanguinis*, **17**, 314–315.

Mead, M. (1939) *From the South Seas*. Vol. 3. *Sex and temperament in three primitive societies*. New York: Morrow.

Meek, C. K. (1925) *The Northern Tribes of Nigeria*. London: Oxford University Press.

Meek, C. K. (1937) *Law and Authority in a Nigerian Tribe. A Study in Indirect Rule*. London: Oxford University Press.

Mercier, P. (1954) The Fon of Dahomey. In *African Worlds* (Ed.) Forde, D. p. 218. London: Oxford University Press.

Messer, J., Willard, D., Kieny, R. & Weitzenblum, S. (1972) Rupture and cardiac embolism of a fragment of an umbilical catheter. Successful surgical removal. *Pédiatrie* (Lyon), **8**, 341–349.

Metrakos, J. D., Metrakos, K. & Baxter, H. (1958) Cleft of the lip and palate in twins. *Plastic and Reconstructive Surgery*, **22**, 109.

Métraux, A. (1946) Twin heroes in South American mythology. *Journal of American Folk-lore*, **59**, 114–123.

Meyer, H. C. (1932) Zur Vererbung der Zwillingsschwangerschaft. *Archiv für Rassen und Gesellschaftsbiologie*, **26**, 387–417.

Meyer, W. C., Keith, L. & Webster, A. (1970) Monoamniotic twin pregnancy with the transfusion syndrome: a case report. *Chicago Medical School Quarterly*, **29**, 42–51.

Michaels, L. (1967) Unilateral ischemia of the fused twin placenta: a manifestation of the twin transfusion syndrome. *Canadian Medical Association Journal*, **96**, 402–405.

Miettinen, M. (1954) On triplets and quadruplets in Finland. *Acta Paediatrica*, **43**, supplement **99**, 9–103.

Miettinen, M. & Grönroos, J. A. (1965) A follow-up study of Finnish triplets. *Annales Paediatriae Fenniae* (Helsinki), **11**, 71–83.

Mijsberg, W. A. (1957) Genetic-statistical data on the presence of secondary oöcytary twins among non-identical twins. *Acta Genetica et Statistica Medica*, **7**, 39–42.

Milham, S. (1964) Pituitary gonadotrophin and dizygotic twinning. *Lancet*, **ii**, 566.

Millis, J. (1959) The frequency of twinning in poor Chinese in the maternity hospital, Singapore. *Annals of Human Genetics*, **23**, 171–174.

Mittler, P. (1970) Biological and social aspects of language development in twins. *Developmental Medicine and Child Neurology*, **12**, 741–757.

Mittler, P. (1971) *The Study of Twins* (*Penguin Science of Behaviour*) (Ed.) Foss, B. M. Harmonsworth, Middlesex: Penguin Books Ltd.

Modan, B., Kallner, H., Modan, M. & Nemser, L. (1968) Differential twinning in Israeli major ethnic groups. *American Journal of Epidemiology*, **88**, 189–194.

Moir, J. C. (1964) *Operative Obstetrics*. London: Bailliere, Tindall and Cox. p. 225.

Moore, N. W. (1973) Ovum development and transfer. *Journal of Reproduction and Fertility*, supplement **18**, 111–116.

Morris, N., Osborn, S. B. & Wright, H. P. (1955) Effective circulation of the uterine wall in late pregnancy measured by ^{24}NaCl. *Lancet*, **i**, 323–324.

Morrison, J. (1974) Personal communication.

Mortimer, B. & Kirschbaum, J. D. (1942) Human double monsters (so-called Siamese twins). *American Journal of Diseases in Childhood*, **64**, 697.

Morton, N. E. (1955) The inheritance of human birthweight. *Annals of Human Genetics*, **20**, 125–134.

Morton, N. E. (1962) Genetics of interracial crosses in Hawaii. *Eugenics Quarterly*, **9**, 23–24.

Morton, N. E. (1970) Birth defects in racial crosses. In *Congenital Malformations* (Ed.) Fraser, F. C. & McKusick, V. A. pp. 264–274. Amsterdam, New York: Excerpta Medica.

Mudaliar, A. L. (1930) Double monsters—the study of their circulatory system and some other anatomical abnormalities and the complications in labour. *Journal of Obstetrics and Gynaecology of the British Empire*, **37**, 753.

Mulligan, T. O. (1970) Personal communication.

Munnell, E. W. & Taylor, H. C. (1946) Complications and fetal mortality in 136 cases of multiple pregnancy. *American Journal of Obstetrics and Gynecology*, **52**, 588–597.

Myrianthopoulos, N. C. (1970) An epidemiologic survey of twins in a large prospectively studied population. *American Journal of Human Genetics* (New York), **22**, 611–629.

Myrianthopoulos, N. W., Churchill, J. A. & Baszynski, A. J. (1971) Respiratory distress syndrome in twins. *Acta Geneticae Medicae et Gemellologiae*, **20**, 199–204.

Naeye, R. L. (1963) Human intrauterine parabiotic syndrome and its complications. *New England Journal of Medicine*, **268**, 804–809.

Naeye, R. L. (1964) The fetal and neonatal development of twins. *Pediatrics* (New York), **33**, 546–533.

Naeye, R. L. (1965) Organ abnormalities in a human parabiotic syndrome. *American Journal of Pathology*, **46**, 829–842.

Naeye, R. L., Benirschke, K., Hagstrom, J. W. C. & Marcus, C. C. (1966). Intrauterine growth of twins as estimated from liveborn birthweight data. *Pediatrics* (New York), **37**, 409–416.

Nance, W. E. (1959) Twins: an introduction to gemellology. *Medicine* (Baltimore), **38**, 403–414.

Napolitani, F. D. & Schreiber, I. (1960) The acardiac monster. A review of the world literature and presentation of two cases. *American Journal of Obstetrics and Gynecology*, **80**, 582–589.

Natelson, S. E. & Sayers, M. P. (1973) The fate of children sustaining severe head trauma during birth. *Pediatrics*, **51**, 169–174.

Nelson, T. R. (1955) A clinical study of pre-eclampsia. *Journal of Obstetrics and Gynaecology of the British Empire*, **62**, 48–66.

Newman, H. H. (1942) Twins and super twins: a study of twins, triplets, quadruplets and quintuplets. In Miettinen, M. (1954) *Acta Paediatrica*, **43**, supplement **99**, 9–103.

Newman, H. H. (1961) *Scientific Monthly*, **52**, 99.

Newman, H. H. & Gardner, I. C. (1942) Types and frequencies of quadruplets: studies of quadruplets. *Journal of Heredity*, **33**, 311–314.

Nichols, B. L., Blattner, R. J. & Rudolph, A. J. (1967) General clinical management of thoracopagus twins. *Birth Defects; Original Article Series* (New York), **3**(1), 38–51.

Nielsen, J. (1967) Inheritance in monozygotic twins. *Lancet*, **ii**, 717–718.

Nissen, E. D. (1958) Twins: collision, impaction, compaction and interlocking. *Obstetrics and Gynecology*, **11**, 154.

Nora, J. J. & Spangler, R. D. (1972) Risks and counselling in cardiovascular malformations. *Birth Defects; Original Article Series* (New York), **8**, 154–159.

Novotny, C. A., Hass, W. K. & Callagan, D. A. (1959) Early diagnosis of multiple pregnancy. Use of electroencephalograph in prenatal examination. *Journal of the American Medical Association*, **171**, 880–884.

Nylander, P. P. S. (1967) Twinning in West Africa. *World Medical Journal*, **14**, 178–180.

Nylander, P. P. S. (1969) The frequency of twinning in a rural community in Western Nigeria. *Annals of Human Genetics*, **33**, 41–44.

Nylander, P. P. S. (1970a) A simple method for determining monochorionic and dichorionic placentation in twins. *Nigerian Journal of Science*, **4**, 239–244.

Nylander, P. P. S. (1970b) The determination of zygosity—a study of 608 pairs of twins born in Aberdeen. *Journal of Obstetrics and Gynaecology of the British Commonwealth*, **77**, 506–510.

Nylander, P. P. S. (1970c) Placental forms and zygosity determination of twins in Ibadan, Western Nigeria. *Acta Geneticae Medicae et Gemellologiae*, **19**, 49–54.

Nylander, P. P. S. (1970d) Twinning in Nigeria. *Acta Geneticae Medicae et Gemellologiae*, **19**, 457–464.

Nylander, P. P. S. (1971a) Biosocial aspects of multiple births. *Journal of Biosocial Science*, supplement **3**, 29.

Nylander, P. P. S. (1971b) Ethnic differences in twinning rates in Nigeria. *Journal of Biosocial Science*, **3**, 151–157.

Nylander, P. P. S. (1971c) The incidence of triplets and higher multiple births in some rural and urban populations in Western Nigeria. *Annals of Human Genetics*, **34**, 409–415.

Nylander, P. P. S. (1973) Serum levels of gonadotrophins in relation to multiple pregnancy in Nigeria. *Journal of Obstetrics and Gynaecology of the British Commonwealth*, **80**, 651.

Nylander, P. P. S. (1974) Personal communication.

Nylander, P. P. S. & Corney, G. (1969) Placentation and zygosity of twins in Ibadan, Nigeria. *Annals of Human Genetics*, **33**, 31–40.

Nylander, P. P. S. & Corney, G. (1971) Placentation and zygosity of triplets and higher multiple births in Ibadan, Nigeria. *Annals of Human Genetics*, **34**, 417–426.

Nylander, P. P. S. & Corney, G. (1975) Placentation and zygosity of twins in Northern Nigeria. In preparation.

Nylander, P. P. S. & Osunkoya, B. O. (1970) Unusual monochorionic placentation with heterosexual twins. *Obstetrics and Gynecology*, **36**, 621–625.

Oettle, A. G. (1953) Paternal influence in polyzygotic births; a family tree with a review of the inheritance of twinning and the paternal mechanisms. *Journal of Obstetrics and Gynaecology of the British Empire*, **60**, 775–784.

Osborne, R. H. & De George, F. V. (1957) Selective survival in dizygotic twins in relation to the ABO blood groups. *American Journal of Human Genetics*, **9**, 321–330.

Ounsted, M. & Ounsted, G. (1973) *On Fetal Growth (its Variations and their Consequences); Clinics in Developmental Medicine No. 46*. Spastics International Medical Publications. London: William Heinemann Medical Books; Philadelphia: J. B. Lippincott Co.

Paintin, D. B. (1962) The size of the total red cell volume in pregnancy. *Journal of Obstetrics and Gynaecology of the British Commonwealth*, **69**, 719–723.

Parkes, A. S. (1969) Multiple births in man. *Journal of Reproduction and Fertility*, supplement **6**, 105–116.

Parmar, V. T. & Mulgund, S. V. (1968) Interlocking of twin pregnancy in uterus circuatus subseptus. *Journal of Postgraduate Medicine*, **14**, 139.

Parrinder, G. (1967) *African Mythology*. London: Hamlyn.

Parsons, P. A. (1964) Birthweights and survival of unlike-sexed twins. *Annals of Human Genetics* (London), **28**, 1–10.

Patten, P. T. (1970) Perinatal mortality by birth order in multiple pregnancy. *Australian and New Zealand Journal of Obstetrics and Gynaecology*, **10**, 27.

Patterson, J. T. (1913)—quoted by Stockard, C. R. (1921) *American Journal of Anatomy*, **28**, 115–277.

Pedlow, P. R. B. (1961) Anencephaly in a mono-amniotic twin. *British Medical Journal*, **ii**, 997.

Pembrey, M. E. (1972) Discordant identical twins. Neural tube defects. *Practitioner*, **209**, 709–712.

Pitt-Rivers, W. R. (1914) *History of Melanesian Society*, Vol. 1. Cambridge: University Press.

Portes, L. & Granjon, A. (1946) Les presentations au cours des accouchments genellaires. *Gynécologie et Obstétrique*, **45**, 1459.

Potter, E. L. (1961) The effect on the foetus of viral disease in the mother. *Clinical Obstetrics and Gynecology*, **4**, 327–340.

Potter, E. L. (1963) Twin zygosity and placental form in relation to the outcome of the pregnancy. *American Journal of Obstetrics and Gynecology*, **87**, 566–577.

Potter, E. L. & Crunden, A. B. (1941) Twin pregnancies in the service of the Chicago Lying-in Hospital. *American Journal of Obstetrics and Gynecology*, **42**, 870–878.

Potter, E. L. & Fuller, H. (1949) Multiple pregnancies at the Chicago Lying-in Hospital, 1941–47. *American Journal of Obstetrics and Gynecology*, **58**, 139–146.

Price, B. (1950) Primary biases in twin studies: review of prenatal and natal difference-producing factors in monozygotic pairs. *American Journal of Human Genetics*, **2**, 293–352.

Prokop, Von O. & Herrmann, U. (1973) Blutgruppenbefunde bei achtlingen. *Zentrablatt für Gynäkologie*, **95**, 1497.

Quigley, J. K. (1935) Monoamniotic twin pregnancy. A case record with a review of the literature. *American Journal of Obstetrics and Gynecology*, **29**, 355.

Race, R. R. & Sanger, R. (1975) *Blood Groups in Man*, 6th edition. Oxford: Blackwell Scientific Publications.

Radasch, H. E. (1921) Superfoetation or superfecundation? *Surgery, Gynecology and Obstetrics*, **32**, 339–352.

Radford, E. & Radford, M. A. (1961) Twins. In *Encyclopaedia of Superstitions* (Ed.) Hole, C. p. 344. London: Hutchinson.

Rausen, A. R., Seki, M. & Strauss, L. (1965) Twin transfusion syndrome. A review of 19 cases studied at one institution. *Journal of Pediatrics*, **66**, 613–628.

Record, R. G., McKeown, T. & Edwards, J. H. (1970) An investigation of the differences in measured intelligence between twins and single births. *Annals of Human Genetics* (London), **34**, 11–20.

Registrar General (1958) *Statistical Review of England and Wales for the year 1956. Part III Commentary*. London: H.M. Stationery Office.

Registrar General (1963–1969) *Statistical Review of England and Wales for the years 1961–1967*. London: H.M. Stationery Office.

Reisner, S. H., Forbes, A. E. & Cornblath, M. (1965) The smaller of twins and hypoglycaemia. *Lancet*, **i**, 524–526.

Revesz, T. (1973) Discordant identical twins: VII Christmas disease. *Practitioner*, **210**, 162–164.

Rice-Wray, E., Cervantes, A., Gutiérrez, J. & Marquez-Monter, H. (1971) Pregnancy and progeny after hormonal contraceptives—genetic studies. *Journal of Reproductive Medicine*, **6**, 101–104.

Roberts, D. F. & Tanner, R. E. S. (1963) Effects of parity on birth weight and other variables in a Tanganyika Bantu sample. *British Journal of Preventive and Social Medicine*, **17**, 209–215.

Robertson, E. G. (1969) Oedema in normal pregnancy. *Journal of Reproduction and Fertility*, supplement **9**, 27.

Robertson, J. G. (1964) Twin pregnancy. Influence of early admission on fetal survival. *Obstetrics and Gynecology*, **23**, 854–860.

Robertson, S. & Grant, A. (1972) Combined intra-uterine and extra-uterine pregnancy in two patients treated with human pituitary gonadotrophins. *Australian and New Zealand Journal of Obstetrics and Gynaecology*, **12**, 253–254.

Robinson, J. S. & Thorburn, G. D. (1974) The initiation of labour. *British Journal of Hospital Medicine*, **12**, 15.

Robinson, R. (1971a) Problems of the newborn: the pre-term baby. *British Medical Journal*, **iv**, 416–419.

Robinson, R. (1971b) Problems of the newborn: the small-for-dates baby. *British Medical Journal*, **ii**, 480–484.

Romanowski, R. (1962) Perinatal mortality in twins. Two year hospital experience. *Bulletin of the Millard Fillmore Hospital*, **9**, 61–71.

Rorie, D. (1914) Stray notes on the folk-lore of Aberdeenshire and the North-east of Scotland. *Folk-lore*, **25**, 342–363.

Ross, R. C. & Philpott, N. W. (1953) Five year survey of multiple pregnancies. *Canadian Medical Association Journal*, **69**, 247–249.

Ross, W. F. (1952) Twin pregnancy in the African. *British Medical Journal*, **ii**, 1336–1337.

Rovinsky, J. J. & Jaffin, H. (1965) Cardiovascular haemodynamics in pregnancy. 1. Blood and plasma volumes in multiple pregnancy. *American Journal of Obstetrics and Gynecology*, **93**, 1–15.

Rovinsky, J. J. & Jaffin, H. (1966a) 2. Cardiac output and left ventricular work in multiple pregnancy. *American Journal of Obstetrics and Gynecology*, **95**, 781–786.

Rovinsky, J. J. & Jaffin, H. (1966b) 3. Cardiac rate, stroke volume, total peripheral resistance and central blood volume in multiple pregnancy. Synthesis of results. *American Journal of Obstetrics and Gynecology*, **95**, 787–794.

Rudolph, A. J., Michaels, J. P. & Nichols, B. L. (1967) Obstetric management of conjoined twins. *Birth Defects; Original Article Series*, **3**(1), 28–37.

Russell, E. M. (1961) Cerebral palsied twins. *Archives of Disease in Childhood*, **36**, 328.

Russell, J. K. (1952) Maternal and fetal hazards associated with twin pregnancy. *Journal of Obstetrics and Gynaecology of the British Empire*, **59**, 209–213.

Sacks, M. O. (1959) Occurrence of anaemia and polycythemia in phenotypically dissimilar single-ovum twins. *Pediatrics*, **24**, 604–608.

Scammon, R. E. (1925) Fetal malformations. In *Pediatrics* (Ed.) Abt, I. A. Vol. 6, p. 654, Philadelphia: Saunders.

Schaffer, A. J. (1963) *Diseases of the Newborn*. Philadelphia, London: Saunders.

Schapera, I. (1927) Customs relating to twins in South Africa. *Journal of the African Society*, **26**, 117–137.

Schatz, F. (1875) Zur Frage über die Quelle des Fruchtwassers und über Embryones papyracei. *Archiv für Gynäkologie*, **7**, 336–338.

Schatz, F. (1882) Eine besondere Art von einseitiger Polyhydramnie mit anderseitiger Oligohydramnie bei eineiigen Zwillingen (Makrocardii). *Archiv für Gynäkologie*, **19**, 329–369.

Schatz, F. (1884) Die Gefässverbindungen der Placentakreisläufe eineiiger Zwillinge, ihre Entwicklung und ihre Folgen. I. Die Gefässverbindungen an der ausgebildeten Placenta. *Archiv für Gynäkologie*, **24**, 337–399.

Schatz, F. (1885) Die Gefässverbindungen der Placentakreisläufe eineiiger Zwillinge, ihre Entwicklung und ihre Folgen. II. Die Entwicklung der Gefässverbindungen und ihre Folgen; A. Die Entwicklung. *Archiv für Gynäkologie*, **27**, 1–72.

Schatz, F. (1887a) Die Gefässverbindungen der Placentakreisläufe eineiiger Zwillinge, ihre Entwicklung und ihre Folgen. II. Die Entwicklung der Gefässverbindungen und ihre Folgen. B. Die Folgen. *Archiv für Gynäkologie*, **29**, 419–442.

Schatz, F. (1887b) Die Gefässverbindungen der Placentakreisläufe eineiiger Zwillinge, ihre Entwicklung und ihre Folgen. II. [Die Folgen: (1) Allgemeiner Theil, (2) Specieller Theil. *Archiv für Gynäkologie*, **30**, 169–240, 335–381.

Schatz, F. (1897–1900) Die Gefässverbindungen der Placentakreisläufe eineiiger Zwillinge, ihre Entwicklung und ihre Folgen. III. Die Acardii und ihre Verwandten. *Archiv für Gynäkologie*, **53**, 144–182; **55**, 485–615; **58**, 1–82; **60**, 81–146; 201–251.

Schatz, F. (1900a) *Klinische Beiträge zur Physiologie des Fötus*. Berlin: Hirschwald.

Schatz, F. (1900b) Systematisches und alphabetisches Inhaltsverzeichniss. *Archiv für Gynäkologie*, **60**, 559–584.

Schatz, F. (1910) Nachträge zu meinem Monograph; Die Gefässverbindungen der Placentakreisläufe eineiiger Zwillinge, ihre Entwicklung und ihre Folgen. *Archiv für Gynäkologie*, **92**, 13–30.

Scheinfeld, A. (1973) *Twins and Supertwins*. London: Penguin Books.

Schinke, R. N., Leape, L. L. & Holder, T. M. (1972) Familial occurrence of oesophageal atresia, a preliminary report. *Birth Defects; Original Article Series*, **8**, 22–23.

Scott, J. M. & Ferguson-Smith, M. A. (1973) Heterokaryotypic monozygotic twins and the acardiac monster. *Journal of Obstetrics and Gynaecology of the British Commonwealth*, **80**, 52–59.

Scott, J. M. & Paterson, L. (1966) Monozygous anencephalic triplets. *Journal of Obstetrics and Gynaecology of the British Commonwealth*, **73**, 147.

Scrimgeour, J. B. & Baker, T. G. (1974) A possible case of superfetation in Man. *Journal of Reproduction and Fertility*, **36**, 69–73.

Sealey, P. V. (1973) Ibeji—the deity of twins among the Yoruba. *Journal of the National Medical Association*, **65**, 443.

Segy, L. (1970) The Yoruba Ibeji statue. *Acta Tropica*, **27**, 97–145.

Severn, C. B. & Holyoke, E. A. (1973) Human acardiac anomalies. *American Journal of Obstetrics and Gynecology*, **116**, 358–365.

Sherman, G. H. & Lowe, E. W. (1970) Do twins carry a high risk for mother and baby? *Journal of the National Medical Association* (New York), **62**, 217–220.

Shipley, P. W., Wray, J. A., Hechter, H. H., Arellano, M. G. & Borhani, N. O. (1967) Frequency of twinning in California: its relationship to maternal age, parity and race. *American Journal of Epidemiology*, **85**, 147–156.

Shorland, J. (1971) Management of the twin transfusion syndrome. *Clinical Pediatrics* (Philadelphia), **10**, 160–163.

Short, R. V. (1970) The bovine free-martin: a new look at an old problem. *Philosophical Transactions of the Royal Society*, Series B, **259**, 141–147.

Simpson, J. S. (1969) Separation of conjoined thoracopagus twins, with the report of an additional case. *Canadian Journal of Surgery* (Toronto), **12**, 89–96.

Škerlj, B. (1939) Cited by Gedda, L. (1961) in *Twins in History and Science*. Springfield, Illinois: Charles C. Thomas.

Smellie, W. (1752) *A Treatise on the Theory and Practice of Midwifery*. Printed for D. Wison at Plato's Head, near Round Court in the Strand, London.

Smith, A. (1974) Observations on the determinants of human multiple birth. *Annual Report of the Registrar General for Scotland, 1964*.

Smith, J. J. & Benjamin, F. (1968) Post haemorrhagic anaemia and shock in the newborn at birth. *Obstetrics and Gynecology*, **23**, 511–521.

Smith, S. M. & Penrose, L. S. (1955) Monozygotic and dizygotic twin diagnosis. *Annals of Human Genetics*, **19**, 273–289.

Smith, W. (1853) *A Smaller Classical Dictionary of Biography, Mythology and Geography*. London: Murray.

Southern, E. M. (1954) Electrocardiography and phonocardiography of the fetal heart. *Journal of Obstetrics and Gynaecology of the British Empire*, **61**, 231–237.

Speke, J. H. (1863) *Journey of the Discovery of the Source of the Nile*. Edinburgh, London: Blackwood.

Spencer, B. & Gillen, F. J. (1899) *The Native Tribes of Central Australia*. London: Macmillan.

Spencer, P. (1965) *The Samburu: a Study of Gerontocracy in a Nomadic Tride*. Los Angeles: University of California Press.

Spurway, J. H. (1962) Fate and management of the second twin. *American Journal of Obstetrics and Gynecology*, **83**, 1377–1388.

Stark, J. (1972) Cardiac surgery in early infancy. *Postgraduate Medical Journal* (London), **48**, 478–485.

Statistical Bulletin of the Metropolitan Life Insurance Company (1960).

Steiner, F. (1935) Nachgeburtsbefund bei Mehrlingen und Anlichkeitsdiagnose. *Archiv für Gynäkologie*, **159**, 509–523.

Stevenson, A. C., Johnston, H. A., Stewart, M. I. P. & Golding, D. R. (1966) Congenital malformations. A report of a study of a series of consecutive births in 24 centres. *Bulletin of the World Health Organization*, **34** (supplement), 1–127.

Stevenson, I. (1941a) Twins among primitive peoples. *Ciba Symposia*, **2**, 702–705.

Stevenson, I. (1941b) Twins as magicians and healing gods: twin myths. *Ciba Symposia*, **2**, 694–701.

Stockard, C. R. (1921) Developmental rate and structural expression: an experimental study of twins, double monsters and single deformities, and the interaction among embryonic organs during their origin and development. *American Journal of Anatomy*, **28**, 115–277.

Strong, S. J. & Corney, G. (1967) *The Placenta in Twin Pregnancy*. Oxford: Pergamon Press.

Studdiford, W. E. (1936) Is superfetation possible in the human being? *American Journal of Obstetrics and Gynecology*, **31**, 845–855.

Sturkie, P. D. (1946) The production of twins in *Gallus domesticus. Journal of Experimental Zoology*, **101**, 51–63.

Sutherland, H. W. & Stowers, J. M. (1975) *Carbohydrate Metabolism in Pregnancy and the Newborn*. Edinburgh, London, New York: Churchill Livingstone.

Sutherland, H. W., Stowers, J. M. & MacKenzie, C. (1970) Simplifying the clinical problem of glycosuria in pregnancy. *Lancet*, **i**, 1069–1071.

Swann, R. O. (1957) Interlocking and collision in multiple pregnancies. Two case reports. *American Journal of Obstetrics and Gynecology*, **73**, 907–910.

Swapp, G. H. (1975) Personal communication.

Szendi, B. (1939) Double monsters in the light of recent biological experiments and investigations regarding heredity. Contribution to the problem of determination of sex. *Journal of Obstetrics and Gynaecology of the British Empire*, **46**, 836–847.

Talbot, P. A. (1926a) *The Peoples of Southern Nigeria*. Vol. 2. London: Oxford University Press. (New impression (1969), London: Cass.)

Talbot, P. A. (1926b) *The Peoples of Southern Nigeria*. Vol. 3. London: Oxford University Press. (New impression (1969), London: Cass.)

TambyRaja, R. L., Anderson, A. B. M. & Turnbull, A. C. (1974) quoted by Robinson, J. S. & Thorburn, G. D. *British Journal of Hospital Medicine*, July, 1974.

Tan, K. L., Goon, S. M., Salmon, Y. & Wee, J. H. (1971a) Conjoined twins. *Acta Obstetrica et Gynecologica Scandinavica*, **50**, 373–380.

Tan, K. L., Tock, E. P. C., Dawood, M. Y. & Ratnam, S. S. (1971b) Conjoined twins in a triplet pregnancy. *American Journal of Diseases of Children*, **122**, 455–458.

Tchouriloff, M. (1877) *Bulletin de la Société d'Anthropologie de Paris*, **12**, 440–446.

Temple, O. (1922) *Notes on the Tribes, Provinces, Emirates and States of the Northern Provinces of Nigeria* (Ed.) Temple, C. L. Lagos: C. M. S. Bookshop.

Templeton, A. & Kelman, R. (1974) Personal communication.

Teoh, E. S., Dawood, M. Y. & Ratnam, S. S. (1970) Epidemiology of hydatidiform mole in Singapore. *American Journal of Obstetrics and Gynecology*, **110**, 415–420.

Theron, J. P. (1969) A case of locked twins in a double uterus. *Journal of Obstetrics and Gynaecology of the British Commonwealth*, **76**, 750.

Thomas, N. W. (1919) Twins. *Man*, **19**, 173–174.

Thomas, N. W. (1921) Twins in the Yoruba country. *Man*, **21**, 140.

Thompson, B. & Baird, D. (1967) Some impressions of childbearing in tropical areas. II. Pre-eclampsia and low birthweight. *Journal of Obstetrics and Gynaecology of the British Commonwealth*, **74**, 499–509.

Timonen, S. & Carpen, E. (1968) Multiple pregnancies and photo-periodicity. *Annales Chirurgiae et Gynaecologiae Fenniae*, **57**, 135–138.

Tow, S. H. (1959) Fetal wastage in twin pregnancy. *Journal of Obstetrics and Gynaecology of the British Empire*, **66**, 444.

Turksoy, R. N., Toy, B. L., Rogers, J. & Papageorge, W. (1967) Birth of septuplets following human gonadotrophin administration in Chiari–Frommel syndrome. *Obstetrics and Gynecology*, **30**, 692–698.

Turpin, R., Bocquet, L. & Grasset, J. (1967) Étude d'un couple monozygote: fille normale—monstre acardiaque féminin. Considerations anatomopathologiques et cytogénétiques. *Annales de Génétique*, **10**, 107–113.

Turpin, R., Lejeune, J., Lafourcade, J., Chigot, P. L. & Salmon, C. (1961) Présomption de monozygotisme en dépit d'un dimorphisme sexuel: sujet masculin et sujet neutre Haplo X. *Comptes Rendus Hebdomadaires des Séances de l'Académie des Sciences*, **252**, 2945–2946.

Vallois, H. V. (1949) La répartition des groupes sanguins en France: l'Ouest armorico-vendéen. *Archiv der Julius Klaus-Stiftung für Vererbungsforschung, Sozialanthropologie und Rassenhygiene*, **24**, 508–516.

Vandeplassche, M., Podliachouk, L. & Beaud, R. (1970) Some aspects of twin-gestation in the mare. *Canadian Journal of Comparative Medicine (and Veterinary Science)*, **34**, 218–226.

Van Der Veen, J. (1972) Hydrodynamics of Holter ventriculoatrial shunt systems under various conditions. *Developmental Medicine and Child Neurology*, **14**, supplement **27**, 132–139.

Veith, I. (1960) Twin birth: blessing or disaster. A Japanese view. *International Journal of Social Psychiatry*, **6**, 230–236.

Verger, P. (1960) Nigeria, Brazil and Cuba. *Nigeria Magazine*, October, 113–123.

Verger, P. (1968) *Flux et Reflux de la Traite des Nègres entre Le Golfe de Bénin et Bahia de Todos os Santos*. Paris: Mouton.

Vestergaard, P. (1972) Triplet pregnancy with a normal foetus and a dicephalus dibrachius sirenomelus. *Acta Obstetrica et Gynecologica Scandinavica*, **51**, 93–94.

Wagner, G. (1936) The study of culture contact and the determination of policy. *Africa*, **9**, 317–331.

Walker, J. & Turnbull, E. P. N. (1955) The environment of the foetus in human multiple pregnancy. *Études néo-natales*, **3**, 123–148.

Walker, J. & Turnbull, E. P. N. (1966) The relationship of the rate of intrauterine growth of infants of low birthweight to mortality, morbidity and congenital anomalies. *Journal of Paediatrics*, **69**, 531–545.

Walker, N. F. (1952) A discussion of the zygosity and asymmetries of two pairs of conjoined twins. *Acta Geneticae Medicae et Gemellologiae*, **1**, 136–151.

Wallace, L. R. (1951) Flushing of ewes. *New Zealand Journal of Agriculture*, **83**, 377–380.

Ward, H., Whyley, G. A. & Miller, M. D. (1972) Serial serum diamine oxidase estimations in normal singleton and twin pregnancies and in abnormal pregnancies. *Journal of Obstetrics and Gynaecology of the British Commonwealth*, **79**, 216–221.

Ware, H. D. (1971) The second twin. *American Journal of Obstetrics and Gynecology*, **110**, 855–873.

Webster, H. (1942) *Taboo. A Sociological Study*. London: Oxford University Press.

Wehefritz, E. (1925) Über die Vererbung der Zwillingsschwangerschaft. *Zeitschrift für Konstitutionslehre*, **11**(2), 554–575.

Weinberg, W. (1902) Beiträge zur Physiologie und Pathologie der Mehrlingsgeburten beim Menschen. *Pflügers Archiv für die gesamte Physiologie des Menschen und der Tiere*, **88**, 346–430.

Weinberg, W. (1909) Die Anlage zur Mehrlingsgeburt beim Menschen und ihre Vererbung. *Archiv für Rassen und Gesellschaftsbiologie*, **6**, 322–339, 470–482, 609–630.

Wenner, R. (1956) Les examens vasculaires des placentas gemellaires et la diagnostic des jumeaux homozygotes. *Bulletin de la Société Royale Belge de Gynécologie et Obstetrique*, **26**, 773–781.

Weyer, E. M. (1932) *The Eskimos. Their Environment and Folkways*. London: Oxford University Press.

Wharton, B., Edwards, J. H. & Cameron, A. H. (1968) Monoamniotic twins. *Journal of Obstetrics and Gynaecology of the British Commonwealth*, **75**, 158–163.

White, C. & Wyshak, G. (1964) Inheritance in human dizygotic twinning. *New England Journal of Medicine*, **271**, 1003.

Wiener, G. (1962) Psychologic correlates of premature birth: a review. *Journal of Nervous and Mental Disease*, **134**, 129–144.

Willerman, L. & Churchill, J. A. (1967) Intelligence and birthweight in identical twins. *Child Development*, **38**, 623–629.

Williams, B. & Cummings, G. (1953) Unusual case of twins: case report. *Journal of Obstetrics and Gynaecology of the British Empire*, **60**, 319–321.

Williams, J. W. (1926) Note on placentation in quadruplet and triplet pregnancy. *Bulletin of the Johns Hopkins Hospital*, **39**, 271–280.

Wilson, E. A. (1972) Holoacardius. *Obstetrics and Gynecology*, **40**, 740–748.

Wilson, R. S., Brown, A. M. & Matheny, A. P. Jr (1971) Emergence and persistence of behavioural differences in twins. *Child Development*, **42**, 1381–1398.

Winer, A. E., Bergman, W. D. & Fields, C. (1957) Combined intra- and extra-uterine pregnancy. *American Journal of Obstetrics and Gynecology*, **74**, 170–178.

Witschi, E. (1970) Teratogenic effects from overripeness of the egg. In *Congenital Malformations* (Ed.) Fraser, F. C. & McKusick, V. A. p. 157. New York: Excerpta Medica.

Wood, C. & Pinkerton, J. H. M. (1966) Uterine activity following the birth of the first twin. *Australian and New Zealand Journal of Obstetrics and Gynaecology*, **6**, 95–99.

Wood, C., Bannerman, R. H., Booth, R. I. & Pinkerton, J. H. M. (1965) The prediction of premature labour by observation of the cervix and external tocography. *American Journal of Obstetrics and Gynecology*, **21**, 396.

Wyshak, G. & White, C. (1963) Birth hazard of the second twin. *Journal of the American Medical Association*, **186**, 869–970.

Wyshak, G. & White, C. (1965) Genealogical study of human twinning. *American Journal of Public Health*, **55**, 1586–1593.

Young, D. G. & Drainer, I. K. (1972) Oesophageal atresia. *British Journal of Hospital Medicine*, **7**, 629–636.

Ysander, F. (1924) A human double embryo of the 6th week. *Uppsala Läkareförenings Förhandlingar*, **29**, 428–434.

Ysander, F. (1925) Human diplo-terata. I. Studies on the morphology and morphogenesis of thoracopagic monsters. *Uppsala Läkareförenings Förhandlingar*, **30**, 319–374.

Yue, S.-J. (1955) Multiple births in cerebral palsy. *American Journal of Physical Medicine*, **34**, 335–341.

Zeleny, C. (1921) The relative numbers of twins and triplets. *Science*, **53**, 262–263.

Zimmerman, A. A. (1967) Embryologic and anatomic considerations of conjoined twins. *Birth Defects; Original Article Series*, 3(1), 18–27.

Zuckerman, H. & Brzezinski, A. (1961) Multiple pregnancies. *Israel Medical Journal*, **20**, 251–258.

Index

Page numbers in *italic* indicate figures